# RESEARCH IN HEALTH CARE SETTINGS

Applied Social Research Methods Series
Volume 14

# Applied Social Research Methods Series

*Series Editor:*
**LEONARD BICKMAN,** Peabody College, Vanderbilt University
*Series Associate Editor:*
**DEBRA ROG,** National Institute of Mental Health

This series is designed to provide students and practicing professionals in the social sciences with relatively inexpensive softcover textbooks describing the major methods used in applied social research. Each text introduces the reader to the state of the art of that particular method and follows step-by-step procedures in its explanation. Each author describes the theory underlying the method to help the student understand the reasons for undertaking certain tasks. Current research is used to support the author's approach. Examples of utilization in a variety of applied fields, as well as sample exercises, are included in the books to aid in classroom use.

*Volumes in this series:*

# RESEARCH IN HEALTH CARE SETTINGS

## Kathleen E. Grady
## Barbara Strudler Wallston

Applied Social Research Methods Series
Volume 14

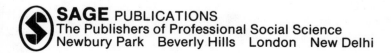

**SAGE** PUBLICATIONS
The Publishers of Professional Social Science
Newbury Park   Beverly Hills   London   New Delhi

*For information address:*

SAGE Publications, Inc.
2111 West Hillcrest Drive
Newbury Park, California 91320

SAGE Publications Inc.
275 South Beverly Drive
Beverly Hills
California 90212

SAGE Publications Ltd.
28 Banner Street
London EC1Y 8QE
England

SAGE PUBLICATIONS India Pvt. Ltd.
M-32 Market
Greater Kailash I
New Delhi 110 048 India

Printed in the United States of America

Library of Congress Cataloging-in-Publication Data

Grady, Kathleen E.
    Research in health care settings.

    (Applied social research methods series; v. 14)
    Bibliography: p.
    Includes index.
    1. Medicine—Research—Methodology.  2. Social
medicine—Research—Methodology.  3. Clinical
health psychology—Research—Methodology.
    I. Wallston, Barbara Strudler.  II. Title.  III. Series.
    R850.G68  1988       362.1′072       88-3154
    ISBN 0-8039-2874-2
    ISBN 0-8039-2875-0 (pbk.)

# CONTENTS

·

# FOREWORD

It is our distinct privilege to write the Foreword for this text. We have had the pleasure of being associated with both Kathy and Barbara prior to their authorship of this volume.

This text is a pioneer in the series as it is the first to focus on a substantive area of research application, rather than on a specific research method. We believe that Kathy and Barbara have not only provided direction to researchers in the health field, but that they have set a high standard for future authors in the series who will have the task of compiling the applied research knowledge for a particular substantive area. This text should be attractive to both the student with little training in research as well as to professionals who need some refreshing on measurement or design. It provides excellent examples and communicates the art of conducting research in health care settings.

The publication of this book is a poignant reminder of Barbara's contributions. Her untimely passing has left a void that continues to be felt by our colleagues in social psychology, health psychology, psychology of women, and the many other fields to which Barbara applied her expertise and skill. This text, one of her last contributions, illustrates Barbara's dedication to societal improvement through high quality research that continues to inspire young and seasoned researchers alike.

—*Debra Rog*
*Leonard Bickman*

# 1

# *Introduction*

Social and behavioral research in health has increased dramatically in recent years. Major shifts in the nature of health and illness have made both the prevention and the management of chronic diseases far more important today than they were a generation ago when the focus of health care was on infectious diseases and acute care (Matarazzo, 1982). There have been major breakthroughs against many infectious diseases, but people are living longer and are more likely to have chronic conditions. In addition, new knowledge about the relationship of risk to disease has led to an increased emphasis on prevention. For both preventing or managing disease, the individual person's behavior and life-style is now recognized as a critical factor. To study this behavior-health link, there is increasing collaboration between social scientists and practicing health professionals in the new areas of behavioral medicine and health psychology. This is the first book on research methods to attempt to speak to both groups and to address the problems and benefits of collaboration between them.

Social and behavioral scientists will recognize the basic research issues discussed in the book. Aspects of the health care system may be unfamiliar to those who have not done health research before, however, and an introduction to the range of possible settings and likely impact on sampling and research design could facilitate the transition to health research. An overview of some of the interpersonal problems may make that transition smoother. Gaining access is an important practical problem and maintaining it can involve ongoing negotiations with health care professionals and systems. There are many ethical issues, some common to research with human subjects and some exacerbated or introduced by the medical aspects of the research, the position of patients, and the doctor-patient relationship. What may attract established researchers are the exciting opportunities for theory-based research with important practical implications.

For the health care professional and student who wishes to do research, our book attempts to provide two things: an abbreviated review of the step-by-step process of conducting research; and a glimpse backstage at the way research is actually done. Real-life examples are shared to illustrate the confusion that experienced researchers know all too well. In addition, we shall discuss the problems of collaboration from the health professional's viewpoint. Training as service providers can make the controlled methods of science seem harsh and insensitive to the concerns of patients. In the press of day-to-day health emergencies, the requirements of data collection can also seem trivial or irrelevant. At the same time, social science collaborators can be overwhelming with their use of jargon, particularly statistics, so that one loses track of the research question or the answer or both.

## MODELS OF RESEARCH

One of the features that distinguishes applied research in general, and health research in particular, is that the research enterprise can start from a variety of vantage points. Sometimes there is a theoretical question to be answered; for example, what are the effects of social support on health and illness? Sometimes a particular health setting will be available for research because that is where one works; for example, a nurse with research interests may be assigned to the intensive care unit. Sometimes a particular sample is the starting point; for example, a pool of patients with the same health problem may become available. The most frequent starting point in health research involves a very practical question with medical significance; examples include the following: How can blood pressure in hypertensive patients be lowered? How can compliance with breast self-examination be increased? What factors influence whether appointments are kept? Where one begins determines what subsequent problems and issues need to be resolved. Perhaps more important is the fact that applied research requires an entirely different model of the research process than the traditional one offered in most textbooks.

### The Traditional Model

The traditional model of research, presented in most standard texts, describes a rational sequence of steps in the process. Research begins with a statement of the problem or research question, backed up by a literature review showing what is already known. Although many texts give little attention to how these questions are actually derived, there is an assumption that in basic research they are derived from theory and in applied research, from a practical problem. The statement of the problem usually ends in the derivation of a specific hypothesis. The method and the sample to be studied are then chosen based on the nature of the question and the extent of existing knowledge. If there has been very little research on the question or phenomenon, more "qualitative" or "developmental" approaches are warranted to provide a more complete description and to develop specific hypotheses. If there has been a substantial amount of research, more "quantitative" methods are recommended with some attention to the relationship of these methods to those previously used. In its narrowest form, the research becomes a "replication and extension" of previous findings. After the study is completed and data collected, data analyses are conducted that are appropriately matched to the design and the kind of data collected. The results are then interpreted in terms of the initial question or problem with passing attention to the limitations of the findings in terms of method and sample. New questions are generated, and it is usually concluded that "further research is needed." This feedback loop makes the overall process circular as well as sequential.

This traditional model of research presents an idealized picture of the process that is far different from how research is *actually* conducted. Robert Merton (1968), a distinguished historian of science, describes the difference between the ideal and the real research process thus:

> [There is a] rockbound difference between scientific work as it appears in print and the actual course of inquiry. . . . The difference is a little like that between textbooks of scientific method and the ways in which scientists actually think, feel, and go about their work. The books on methods present ideal patterns, but these tidy, normative patterns . . . do not reproduce the typically untidy, opportunistic adaptations that scientists really make. The scientific paper presents an immaculate appearance which reproduces little or nothing of the intuitive leaps, false starts, mistakes, loose ends, and happy accidents that actually cluttered up the inquiry.

## The Garbage Can Model

Martin (1982) has presented a competing model that attempts to capture some of the chaos of actual research. She calls hers the "Garbage

Can Model of Research." It is derived from a model of organizational decision making that was also a reaction to the conventional, normative, rational assumptions of how organizations function (Cohen, March, & Olsen, 1972). In Martin's model, four elements swirl about in the garbage can or decision space of the particular research project. These elements are theories, methods, resources, and solutions. Resources include the abilities of the researchers, subject pool, access to field sites, and funds. Solutions include both the results of the data analysis and the interpretation of those results. The key to Martin's model is not the creation of these elements, but their interdependence and co-equal status in the model. Each influences the others and each is a major factor in the outcome of the research. For example, in the traditional model, resources are assigned a passive role; they are merely the conditions that enable research to be conducted. In Martin's model, resources may "function actively, as a determining factor in the selection of a theoretical problem, the choice of a method, and even the interpretation of a solution" (p. 26). Priorities of funding agencies, availability of certain kinds of expertise on the research team, and computer time or programs are resources that can influence other elements in the model.

The Garbage Can Model not only dispenses with the assumption about the sequence of steps in the research process, it also discards the assumption that there is necessarily a feedback loop between solutions and problems. The final data may fail to confirm the initial hypothesis and, moreover, may show some surprising and interesting unanticipated effects. As Martin points out, Skinner (1956, p. 32) serendipitously discovered the first principles of behaviorism as an unanticipated outcome of a research project that had only a vague initial theoretical focus. The search for post hoc explanations for interesting findings may horrify traditional experimental researchers. It is, however, a common state of affairs, particularly in complicated, large-scale, longitudinal research projects.

## Garbage Can II

Health behavior and health care research projects are more likely to be such complicated research projects, involving a team of experts from different fields, a variety of outcomes, and extensive resource requirements. The position adopted in this book is an elaborated version of the Garbage Can Model. Not only theories but problems and phenomena are included in the first element. Nontheoretical sources of research questions, such as personal concerns of the researcher, which Martin specifically excludes, are included. Experimental, quasi-experimental, and nonexperimental designs are touched on. Methods include choosing and integrating measures for several questions and using multiple measures, a common practice in health research. The very important role of resources is acknowledged in terms of expertise, settings, samples, and measures and in terms of identifying and assembling needed resources, evaluating existing resources, and responding to resource opportunities as they arise. Flexible data analytic approaches and a variety of interpretations of findings for different audiences provide a much looser definition of solutions. At the same time, the organization and order of the chapters generally follow the traditional research model but without the same prescription for sequencing. This order should facilitate reference to other standard texts for more detail as needed. The overall model of the research process, whether traditional or Garbage Can, only provides a schema, a broad outline. As the research is actually undertaken, additional complexities become apparent.

<h2 style="text-align:center">RESEARCH IN THE<br>REAL WORLD</h2>

### Judgment Calls

Once a research project has been adequately designed with a well-specified question, methods and samples chosen, and other necessary resources assembled, the assumption generally is that the data collection phase will smoothly unfold. Not so. As one experienced researcher writes:

> There is more to doing research than is dreamt of in philosophies of science, and texts in methodology offer answers to only a fraction of the problems one encounters. The best laid research plans run up against unforeseen contingencies in the collection and analysis of data; the data one collects may prove to have little to do with the hypothesis one sets out to test; unexpected findings inspire new ideas. No matter how carefully one plans in advance, research is designed in the course of its execution. The finished monograph is the result of hundreds of decisions, large and small, made while the research is underway and our standard texts do not give us procedures and techniques for making those decisions. (Becker, 1965, p. 602)

A Nobel laureate in immunology, Sir Peter Medawar goes one step further: "It is no use looking to scientific 'papers,' for they do not merely conceal but actively misrepresent the reasoning which goes into the work they describe" (Judson, 1980, p. 3).

If one cannot learn these decision-making processes from standard textbooks or scientific reasoning from research reports, how does one learn how to do research? Martin (1982, p. 19) has some ideas:

> Students trying to learn how to do research are constantly faced with gaps between the rational model of many of their texts and teachers and the realities of how research actually is conducted. They must learn the "street smarts" of the research process, the rules of thumb that guide practical research decisions. Many students whose classes and textbooks are restricted to the rational approach are forced to learn about the inaccuracies of the rational model in a haphazard fashion. They decipher rules of thumb from throwaway lines in conversations with faculty, asides in methodology textbooks, and embarrassed footnotes in journal articles.

McGrath and his colleagues (1982) call these important and ubiquitous decisions during the conduct of the research "judgment calls." As in baseball, from which the term is borrowed, judgment calls are necessary and cumulative in their consequences so that they can quite literally determine the outcome of the baseball game or the research project. These experienced researchers explicitly reject the notion that such judgment calls should be replaced by more formal decision rules:

> One loses a great deal when one attempts to fashion sound research entirely on the basis of general decision rules routinely applied. Rather, we believe one should retain a very important place for the judgments of the skilled researcher who, at best, will be sensitive to nuances of both the substantive setting and the research impedimenta; and who, at least, can observe when something stunningly unexpected occurs, and can perhaps stop the churning of the research machine long enough to take a look at it. ... At [these] junctures the investigators' unique skills/resources/purposes can be brought to bear. (McGrath et al., 1982, p. 14)

## Hanging Loose

In addition to good judgment, coping with change also requires flexibility, creativity, and the ability to break one's "set" of how things were supposed to proceed and try alternatives. An interesting example comes from the insect world but has been applied by Weick (1981, pp. 3-4) in discussing organizational change:

If you place in a bottle half a dozen bees and the same number of flies, and lay the bottle down horizontally, with its base to the window, you will find that the bees will persist, till they die of exhaustion or hunger, in the endeavor to discover an issue through the glass; while the flies, in less than two minutes, will all have sallied forth through the neck on the opposite side. . . . It is their [the bees'] love of light, it is their very intelligence, that is their undoing in this experiment. They evidently imagine that the issue from every prison must be there where the light shines clearest; and they act in accordance, and persist in too logical action. To them glass is a supernatural mystery they never have met in nature; they have had no experience of this suddenly impenetrable atmosphere; and, the greater their intelligence, the more inadmissible, more incomprehensible, will the strange obstacle appear. Whereas the feather-brained flies, careless of logic as of the enigma of crystal, disregarding the call of the light, flutter wildly hither and thither, and meeting here the good fortune that often waits on the simple, who find salvation there where the wise will perish, necessarily end by discovering the friendly opening that restores their liberty to them.

Wieck concludes, "This episode speaks of experimentation, persistence, trial and error, risks, improvisation, the one best way, detours, confusion, rigidity and randomness all in the service of coping with change." The bees are smarter than the flies but too rigid in their knowledge to respond to novelty.

Throughout this book, we provide examples of real judgment calls made during the conduct of research in order to try to transfer some of the "street smarts" of experienced researchers. The good researcher should have not only the intelligence of bees acquired through knowledge of the rules but also the experimental courage (or desperation) of the flies to be able to respond to novelty and change.

### Making Mistakes

"Experimentation is the fundamental tool of science: if we experiment successfully, by definition, we will make many mistakes" (Peters & Waterman, 1982, p. 48). All researchers make mistakes. In research and development in industry, making mistakes is encouraged and valued as an important way to learn and develop creativity. As one captain of industry tells his workers, "Make sure you generate a reasonable number of mistakes" (Dowling & Byrom, 1978). Peters and Waterman, in their book on excellence in organizations, consider this encouragement one of the characteristics of a successful organization. They cite one company that not only encourages mistakes but celebrates them. They shoot off a cannon every time a "perfect failure" occurs.

> The perfect failure concept arises from simple recognition that all research and development is inherently risky, that the only way to succeed at all is through lots of tries, that management's primary objective should be to induce lots of tries, and that a good try that results in some learning is to be celebrated even when it fails. As a by-product, they legitimize and even create positive feelings around calling a quick halt to an obviously failing proposition, rather than letting it drag on with resulting higher cost in funds and eventual demoralization. (Peters & Waterman, 1982, p. 69)

In contrast, in academia, failures are not publicized. According to McGuire (1983), what tends to be published is a "sanitized version of research, the well-done demonstration of the confirmed hypothesis," which leaves hidden "the greater and more informative part of the process," the mistakes. Typically, a researcher sets up a study to confirm a hypothesis. When the results don't come out "right"—that is, they don't confirm the hypothesis—procedures are reevaluated and changed. If the study never "works," it is never published. If it finally does "work," it is that final study that is written up for publication. Should a researcher ever submit the whole story, editors might suggest, says McGuire (p. 15), "that the researcher's intellectual odyssey in the course of meandering toward the actual experiment may be very interesting to her or his mother but the space crunch in the journal hardly makes it appropriate for publication."

## Fundamental Dilemmas

McGrath (1982) characterizes the research process as inherently a series of problems and choices or dilemmas. He calls this description "dilemmatics" and declares that there is no "dilemmagic" that will make the problems go away. All research methods are inherently flawed, and it is the task of the researcher to acknowledge these flaws and to balance them overall in the acquisition of knowledge. Strategies, designs, and methods must be evaluated in terms of the basic three-horned dilemma of research: the need to maximize (a) generalizability with respect to populations, (b) precision in control and measurement of variables, and (c) existential realism for the participants. Each choice in the research process involves a compromise among two or more of these criteria. For example, laboratory experiments have maximum precision in the control and measurement of variables but lack existential realism for the participants. In addition, the difficulty of enticing a representative sample of the population into a laboratory frequently creates low generalizability with respect to populations. Moving to field experiments increases realism but sacrifices measurement precision and maintains problems of generalizability. Sample surveys have maximum generalizability to populations but only a modest amount of precision and little realism.

According to McGrath, the research process is to be regarded not as a set of problems to be "solved," but rather as a set of dilemmas to be "lived with." Each research project is "poor" in some sense. Something had to be sacrificed in the design or method or sampling. The only way to build knowledge is to do lots of research using various means *that do not share the same weaknesses* (p. 80). Although every researcher cannot be an expert in every kind of research, the intellectual community as a whole can take some responsibility for extending and replicating findings by performing differently flawed research.

### Flawed, Good Research

Recognizing that all research is flawed does not mean that the distinction between "good" and "bad" research has been lost (McGrath, 1982). Bad research is using a method badly and is never acceptable. Failing to understand or to make explicit the flaws in a research method is still bad research. A poor idea, poorly executed, is, as computer buffs say, "Garbage in; garbage out." There is still plenty of room for criticism of research, and there is lots of research that deserves robust criticism. McGrath (1982, p. 102) defines "good research" as using flawed methods well and in effective combinations. Good research can help us accrue knowledge about problems that are of both theoretical and practical concern.

## STYLE AND
## ORGANIZATION OF THE BOOK

### Use of Examples

Throughout the book, we have endeavored to give some flavor of research in the real world by using "backstage" examples based on our own research. It has taken some courage to share with the reader the negotiations, the confusion, the serendipity, and the patchwork solutions we have sometimes employed. Because we have conferred about study problems for many years, we have adopted the pronoun *we* when referring to study examples, although all our research has been done in close collaboration with other colleagues. We also refer to the reader as *you*. This informality deliberately breaks the rules about scientific writing style in a further attempt to demystify the scientific research process.

To understand some of the decision-making processes and the examples used, it may be helpful to know more about us and our research. We are both social psychologists trained in experimental and survey techniques. As social psychologists, we are interested in the characteristics of both people and environments and the complex interactions between them. We have each done health-related research for more than 10 years. A brief description of two lines of research from which several examples are drawn may illustrate some of the differences between us and provide an introduction for the examples.

The research on breast self-examination (BSE) is Grady's. In a series of experiments, several methods for increasing the practice of BSE have been tested. These methods are based on the principles of behavior modification and include increasing the stimulus cues (reminders) for BSE, adding rewarding outcomes for doing BSE, and attempting to "desensitize" women about their fears of BSE. Studies used both patient populations and community samples followed for one to two years to monitor the frequency of BSE when each of these methods was employed. In addition, information about attitudes, behavior, social networks, and many other personal characteristics was collected to determine whether different methods were more successful with certain kinds of women.

The research on health locus of control and choice are Wallston's. The Multidimensional Health Locus of Control Scales (MHLC) consist of three scales that measure whether people perceive the locus (place, point) of control over health outcomes within themselves, in powerful others like physicians and other health professionals, or in fate, luck, or chance. The theory is that different perceptions of locus of control may lead to different behavior and ultimately different health outcomes. Exerting some actual control over aspects of medical care may also affect health outcomes, a hypothesis that was tested in two studies.

Patients being given chemotherapy or about to undergo a noxious medical procedure (barium X-ray) were given choices about aspects of their medical treatment, choices that were not medically significant but could be psychologically significant in that they increased the patient's sense of control. The extent to which patients then had physical or psychological reactions to the treatments was assessed.

## Overall Organization

Because the model of research suggested here is Garbage Can II, where all research elements swirl around in a decision space simultaneously, the organization of the book presented some problems. Which element one begins with in research determines which issues remain to be considered. The order of the chapters, therefore, could be completely arbitrary. Ideally, one should be able to pick up a methods book such as this and read the chapters in the order needed. Unfortunately, writing is linear and it is difficult to present material without a logical sequence. Recognizing the essential arbitrariness of the ordering, we shall follow the traditional model of problem definition, design, sample selection, measurement, conduct of the study, and interpretation. We shall begin with a chapter on health care settings and interdisciplinary team-building, however, because that is perhaps the most distinguishing characteristic of health care research.

## SUMMARY

This book is written for both social scientists and health professionals who wish to do research in health care. A model of research is adopted that reflects the needs of large interdisciplinary research projects. It gives co-equal status to the many elements required by such projects. Experienced researchers are able to adopt an orderly but flexible approach to the research process. There are fundamental dilemmas and limitations in any single research effort. Knowledge is accrued by attacking the same problem using different methods that do not share the same weaknesses. Throughout the book, examples are provided of attempts to cope with problems that arise during the course of research.

# 2

## Health Care Settings and Collaborative Research

A doctor's office is often the first place that comes to mind in thinking of health care settings. It may be a small office in a home or a large group practice in an office building or medical center. It may be one of the new walk-in, 24-hour centers. The dominant image, however, is of a private physician delivering personal care for a medical problem.

While this image is certainly valid, it is only part of the total picture. Health care can be defined much more broadly to encompass a range of services that take place in a variety of settings and are delivered by many kinds of professionals. These settings include physicians' offices; hospitals; clinics; health maintenance organizations (HMOs); nursing homes and other chronic care facilities; voluntary health associations like the American Cancer Society, the Heart Association, and the Ostomy Society; and other workplace and community settings. Health care services include education as well as diagnosis, treatment, prevention, early detection, and rehabilitation. Health care is delivered to groups or individuals and by pamphlets, video, and computer programs as well as by private instruction and prescription. It involves not only physicians but nurses and nurse practitioners, midwives, physical therapists, clinical dietitians, medical technologists and technicians, psychologists, occupational therapists, health educators, dental hygienists, radiology technicians, and other allied health professionals.

Most health care settings offer fruitful possibilities for social and behavioral research. In this chapter, some of the features that distinguish various settings and their implications for research are reviewed. What is the primary purpose of the health care delivered in various settings? How do the populations of patients differ by setting? Also covered in this chapter are issues related to being an "outsider," specifically problems of system entry and maintenance. How does a behavioral scientist new to health research gain access to one of these settings and maintain it? "Insiders," that is health care professionals who want to conduct research, also have problems, in particular, conflicts between their usual clinical role and the research role they wish to undertake.

What are these role conflicts and how can they be minimized? Finally, we discuss the research team. How is one formed and what are the pitfalls and pleasures of collaboration?

## FEATURES OF THE SETTINGS

### Primary Purpose

A major distinction between health care settings is whether they are focused on *illness* or *wellness*. Most health care settings are oriented to illness-care. Many are likely to focus on specific episodes of illness, ranging from heart attacks and broken legs to muscle spasms and the common cold. Emergency rooms exemplify this kind of treatment. This *acute care* orientation may be contrasted to *chronic care*. Because the population of the United States is aging and because there have been dramatic successes in combating infectious diseases, chronic health problems are becoming the focus of increasingly large segments of the health care profession. Nursing homes and the Visiting Nurses Association are oriented to chronic, long-term care. Chronic care may involve *rehabilitation,* for example, from a stroke, or *coping* with irreversible aspects of a health condition like chronic obstructive pulmonary disease. Self-help groups, often sponsored by voluntary health associations, focus on problems of chronic conditions for both patients and family members. Such groups provide an opportunity for people to meet on a regular basis for mutual support and information-sharing about topics such as breast cancer, Alzheimer's disease, brain injuries, or alcoholism.

In addition to the trend toward more chronic care, there is growing attention to wellness, including *disease prevention* and *health promotion*. Work sites increasingly are providing screening and health promotion by offering employees blood pressure testing, exercise opportunities, and weight loss programs. Health fairs are becoming commonplace, and videos and books promoting good nutrition and exercise are best-sellers. To some extent, the promotion of good health habits has always had a place in health care. Dentistry is an example of a health care profession that has long had a major focus on prevention. Voluntary health associations like the American Cancer Society and the American Heart Association have extensive public education programs for prevention and early detection of these major diseases.

It is clear, however, that there is a new and more widespread emphasis on health promotion. Among the many factors that have contributed to this change are the accumulating information about *risk factors* for various diseases and changing *economic factors* in health care delivery. Risk factors have helped identify particular groups of people who should take specific actions to avoid a disease or condition for which they are at risk. For example, it is recommended that DES daughters should undergo regular screening and that people with high cholesterol levels should watch their diets. An economic incentive for prevention has occurred with the establishment of health maintenance organizations (HMOs). They provide all needed medical services for a flat annual fee rather than the traditional fee-for-service where each visit and service is billed separately. The economic incentive for these HMOs then is to keep their patients as well as possible, cutting down on the number of visits and services in order to make a profit within the flat rate fee structure.

The distinctions between a focus on chronic and acute care and illness and wellness are not always perfectly clear. There are chronic diseases, like rheumatoid arthritis, that "flare" or have acute episodes. An acute illness can require surgery followed by lengthy rehabilitation or chronic care. Screening of healthy populations can lead to the detection of a chronic disease, and ill-advised self-help programs, such as "crash" diets, can bring on illness. Because of these relationships, virtually every setting has at least some focus on both illness and wellness. Nonetheless, the distinction is useful for characterizing the major purpose of a health setting, which can determine what kinds of people are likely to be found there and why.

## Population

To a great extent, the setting has already preselected the sample for the researcher. It is well established that people who receive medical care are not representative of the general population. People who go to the doctor are more likely to be women, more likely to be under 5 or over 75 years of age, have a very low or relatively high income, and be white and better educated (U.S. Bureau of the Census, 1985). Within these categories, there are also differences among people with identified diagnoses of illness, those who have symptoms and seek diagnosis, and those who receive routine checkups and preventive care. Most people with diagnosed serious, chronic illness are receiving some kind of health care, but only some people with symptoms seek medical evaluation. Fewer still utilize preventive health care. Only 8% of physician visits are for general checkups whereas 84% are for diagnosis or treatment of conditions.

Of the *sociodemographic* characteristics that influence *medical utilization*, the most obvious discriminating factor is economic. Private health care can be extremely expensive. Much of this cost is covered by medical insurance, and 61% of Americans are covered by insurance through employers (U.S. Bureau of the Census, 1985). Another 10% are covered by public insurance like Medicaid, which is available for poor people, and Medicare, which is available for the elderly. Outside of the medical insurance system entirely are 15% of Americans, including a growing number of recently unemployed and recently divorced. What services and what service providers are covered by insurance has a powerful effect on who is found in what kind of setting. Few insurance policies cover routine office visits, screening, or prevention. At the same time, most insurance policies cover surgery and diagnostic tests. Thus, given customary insurance coverage, prevention and screening can be more expensive to the individual than diagnosis and treatment. It is not the *actual costs* but the *out-of-pocket* expenses that often determine which health services will be sought.

In considering costs that influence health care utilization, it is important to take into account *hidden costs* and costs that are not strictly monetary—*opportunity costs*. Hidden costs would include public transportation and/or parking, and the costs of baby-sitting or respite care for elderly or ill dependents. Opportunity costs refer to the loss of ability to do other things while receiving medical treatment. The most obvious example is the loss of ability to work and earn wages. The amount of time lost can be influenced by the time of day of the program or appointment, the length of time including waiting time, and the length of the program or number of visits needed for treatment. These kinds of related costs can have a differential impact on certain groups of people, such as employed versus unemployed, people with children, or the handicapped.

Another important factor that influences who frequents which setting is *referral patterns*. Many types of health services, particularly medical specialties, require a general practice physician to refer the patient for diagnosis or treatment. A common example would be an internist referring a patient to a surgeon. Referral patterns may influence health care in less obvious ways, however. For example, it has been standard practice until very recently for radiologists to require a referral in order to perform a mammogram. Now, in some places, self-referral or "walk-in" appointments are possible. It is likely that these different referral requirements would influence which women would be getting mammograms in two otherwise identical radiological services. Physician referrals are also necessary for most rehabilitative services. Even the American Cancer Society's "Reach for Recovery" program usually requires a physician referral for a volunteer who has had a mastectomy to contact a woman who has recently undergone the surgery to offer support and advice.

## Impact on Research

Features of the setting such as its purpose and population must be considered when undertaking a research project. They influence virtually every aspect of the study: what types of questions may reasonably be asked, the design of the study, sampling, measures, the conduct of the study, and the inferences that can be drawn from the results. While features of the setting may constrain research, an attempt to understand the setting may contribute to more meaningful research results. Table 2.1 summarizes the features of health care settings discussed so far. It is by no means exhaustive. It does suggest, however, the variety of factors that should be taken into account when evaluating a setting for research purposes.

Settings should be evaluated for the study populations available within them. If one wanted to study health habits among the elderly, different types of settings are likely to be used for treating different segments of the elderly population. Work sites could be excluded as they are unlikely to have many people over 65. Golden Age Clubs are likely to have healthier elderly people participating in their activities. Nursing homes would have the sickest and least independent elderly population. Meal programs at community centers would attract mobile elderly while "meals-on-wheels" would cater to house-bound elderly. Each of these settings and related populations would affect which health habits could be studied, how the study should be conducted, and what inferences may be drawn.

Some settings are inappropriate for certain questions. If one wanted to study smoking cessation, a site with a major focus on preventive health care such as an HMO or a health club would not be a good choice.

TABLE 2.1
Features of a Setting

1. Type
    private physician office
    HMO
    hospital
    nursing home
    health association
    work site
    other community setting

2. Primary Purpose
    illness
        acute care
        chronic care
    wellness
        prevention
        screening
    not health related
        employment
        recreation/leisure
        other focus

3. Population
    sex
    age
    race
    income
    level of illness

4. Cost
    price of service
        insurance coverage
        out-of-pocket cost
    hidden costs
        transportation
        baby-sitting
        lost wages
        other opportunity costs
    factors affecting opportunity costs
        time of day
        length of time for program/appointment
        waiting time
        length of program/number of visits

5. Referral Pattern
    referral needed
        from whom?
    referral not needed

Both the facility and the people who use it are more interested in prevention and health promotion than the population at large. Clients probably are drawn from a segment of the population that is most likely to have never smoked, to have given it up, or to be highly motivated to give it up. Any successes experienced with this population are unlikely to be generalizable (applicable) to most smokers. A preferable alternative for a smoking cessation study might be a work site, a setting that offers a population that has not been prescreened in a manner related to the outcome of interest.

The services and staff in different settings also affect research possibilities. There may be conflicts with planned interventions because of existing procedures or other programs. Interviews may not be feasible because of time or space constraints. Related data may already be routinely collected, or, for other reasons, the research question may be of no interest to the staff. Study procedures may be perceived as a burden by the staff. A thorough knowledge of the setting, its service priorities, and its methods of functioning is a necessary prerequisite for designing and conducting the research. Questions and issues can be developed by reference to the setting features outlined in Table 2.1, but only on-site personnel can provide the answers.

## "OUTSIDER" ISSUES: GAINING AND MAINTAINING ACCESS

Researchers who are not part of the setting in which they wish to conduct research are "outsiders" who must become familiar with aspects of the health care setting or organization that can facilitate entry and cooperation. Settings vary in their openness to research. Some health care facilities have research as an additional goal. The primary example is university-affiliated hospitals that usually have research as part of their mandate. Voluntary health associations are also often open to research because they have programs that need to be evaluated. New HMOs sometimes encourage research to develop their marketing strategy; they need to know who is using their services and which services are most popular. The outside researcher needs to be aware of how research matches the priorities of the organization as well as the decision-making structure, formal and informal, which provides research access.

## Decision-Making Structure

Size is a key feature. Larger settings tend to have more complex decision-making structures. In order to have research approved, there are more levels of approval. There may be a regulatory committee overseeing research. Although all hospitals may seem alike to the outsider, the type of hospital may have different organizational structures that affect patient access. Physicians in a university-affiliated hospital usually have a faculty position. Approaching department heads is often a successful way to enlist the cooperation of these physicians. Sometimes the department head can give permission for access to the patients. In general hospitals, on the other hand, patient access needs to be negotiated with individual physicians who have substantially more control over their private patients.

While most often the physician has formal control over access to patient populations, persons dealing with the patient on a day-to-day basis, such as nurses, technicians, and receptionists, can be critically important in facilitating or hindering real access. The ongoing interpersonal relationships among these health care personnel, the patients, and the physicians may involve subtle power dynamics. Recognizing these informal structures and initiating communication are significant research tasks. The details of the recruitment strategy and methods of data collection must be negotiated with all relevant personnel. Early involvement of such personnel in decision making can improve the research in several ways: (1) by using the information and ideas they may have; (2) by minimizing disruptions to their routines, and (3) by creating a sense of involvement and participation in the research process. While the specific key people may be different in each health care setting, the principle of working with those who have direct contact with study participants holds across settings. Example 2.1 describes a hard-won lesson in involving the right people.

---

*Example 2.1.*
*Taking a Dental Hygienist to Lunch*

In a study designed to predict preventive dental behavior, the cooperation of the private practice dentist was easy to achieve. He was in fact extremely enthusiastic about the research. The research methods, however, required that the receptionist hand out forms to patients to complete while they were in the waiting room and that the hygienist rate each patient's behavior after their visit. The dentist had no actual role in the research. Early in the study, it became apparent that there was a problem. Data collection was incomplete, and the ratings were remarkably similar across patients and not usable for data analysis. The researchers took the receptionist and the dental hygienist to lunch to discuss the basic purposes of the study and their specific roles. Respecting their input and establishing ongoing communication improved the data collection process immediately and permanently.

---

*Strategies for obtaining physician cooperation* are important in almost all health care settings. Why should a busy physician cooperate with your research? You have to communicate to the physician a cost-benefit ratio that will help her or him to decide to cooperate. In order to do this, there are several steps you can take:

(1) You may be interested in a theoretical question but for purposes of presentation to the physician, you need to do some concrete thinking about the *practical and clinical relevance* of your research. What does it have to do with the patient's health or with improving clinical practice? In order to emphasize clinical relevance, however, you do not have to become a medical expert yourself. The doctor is the doctor.

(2) It may facilitate access to have a medically knowledgeable person as a member of the research team. *Collaboration* with physicians and / or nurses can be quite effective. Their knowledge of the health care setting and the clinical activity allows them to converse in a medical setting as one clinician to another. Their presence is also living proof that the research is of interest to clinicians, thereby bolstering your argument for practical and clinical relevance.

(3) Some physicians are interested in cooperating with research projects because there are real *personal benefits* to be gained. They may be interested in the results because they will yield information that improves services. They may want or need scientific publication to further their own career goals. Cooperating for publication credit could involve providing the physician co-authorship on the work or access to the data to ask additional questions of interest. It is important to negotiate issues of authorship early in the process. One should be aware that norms for receiving authorship are different in different fields so it is good to make as few assumptions as possible. Agree about first authorship as well as who will have what level of authorship on which kinds of publications. (See Chapter 10 for further discussion of these issues.)

(4) It helps to have a *clear plan* that includes precisely what is wanted from the physician. Having a brief written summary of the project can

be helpful. Time lines, although sometimes difficult to project and necessarily tentative, can add concreteness to the request. The research should be designed to entail minimum disruption of services. Because space is often scarce, you should be reasonable in making your request. It is important to be flexible and to be willing to compromise around procedures. State your request clearly and in writing. Put the final agreement in writing.

(5) Where significant amounts of staff time are being used, some form of *compensation* may be worked out. A funded research project might purchase some percentage of staff time. Alternately, research staff who are appropriately trained may provide service delivery in addition to or as part of their research tasks. (See example 2.2.)

---

*Example 2.2.*
*Free Help for the Clinic*

A research project on decreasing emesis (vomiting) after chemotherapy needed a chemotherapy nurse to administer the medication and to collect data. Hospital staff were overworked and could spare no time for either research training or data collection. The project was at first viewed as a potential burden on scarce resources despite the fact that there were funds to compensate the clinic for staff time. Project participants were scattered among the regular chemotherapy patients so that on some days there would be several and on other days there would be none. The project decided to hire the needed chemotherapy nurse on a regular part-time basis. When she had no project participants, the hospital clinic was able to use her to provide chemotherapy for other patients. The potential burden was transformed into a benefit for the clinic, enhancing cooperation and allowing data collection to proceed smoothly.

---

## "INSIDER" ISSUES:
## ROLE CONFLICT

Health professionals who are part of the setting in which they wish to conduct research are "insiders" who must step back and view objectively the setting and their usual role within it. There are some inherent conflicts between the role of researcher and the role of clinician. Research requires objectivity, evenhandedness, and controls in terms of treatment. Patient care requires flexibility, sensitivity, and responsiveness to the individual needs of the patient. There are built-in conflicts between these role responsibilities. The health care professional researcher may act differently to subjects in different treatment conditions because she or he is supportive of one kind of treatment and not another. Ethical and professional standards of behavior may be at odds.

## Strategies for Minimizing Role Conflicts

There are things you can do to try to control the inherent role conflicts between health professional and researcher. On occasion, it may require choosing a different research problem or a different method. More commonly, it requires acknowledgment of the problem and acceptable procedural adjustments to control for it.

(1) *Try to foresee* what conflicts are likely to arise in the study. For example, in a study on the effects of drug and alcohol abuse by pregnant teenagers, baseline data needed to be collected about the extensiveness of such substance abuse. Using a structured interview, the researcher asked a series of questions about the young woman's behavior. It was crucial to the integrity of the data that the interviewer not show negative reactions to these responses even though she had enough medical knowledge to realize that some of these behaviors could have very serious consequences for the young woman as well as the fetus. The conflict between the roles of researcher and helping professional was a personal agony for the researcher.

Similarly, in the breast self-examination (BSE) study, we asked respondents to record on the BSE Record any breast changes they found during their examinations and in particular to note any of a list of suspicious changes (lumps, discharge, and so on). As researchers, we were interested in several questions: Did BSE lead to such findings? Which findings prompted a medical evaluation? Which women sought such an evaluation? Were there any delays between finding a change and seeking an evaluation? As people interested in health care, however, we were concerned that any suspicious findings be medically evaluated as promptly as possible. Clinically, we know that early detection and treatment are crucial for breast cancer. Which role was going to dictate how we responded to this information about findings? The conflict was inherent in the study.

(2) *Make a plan* for dealing with possible role conflicts. In the BSE study, we realized that the study participants may be even more confused about our role than we were. Some of them might think that by noting a suspicious finding on their BSE forms, they were going to receive a medical evaluation, that if it were anything truly serious, someone would tell them what to do. We, therefore, decided to adopt a

procedure that would clarify role responsibilities. We developed a letter that was sent whenever a finding was reported on a Record. It reminded the woman that it was up to her to see a doctor of her choice and at her own expense to have the change evaluated. In the substance abuse study, the lack of a response to the information provided by the young women also was considered a possible source of confusion. Respondents might assume that it was all right to continue to abuse drugs or that there was no medical/psychological help available. A procedure was developed to provide appropriate referrals at the end of the interview session, after the baseline study data were collected.

(3) *Record responses* as potential additional variables. If you have foreseen a potential problem, you can standardize a plan for dealing with it and record that it has been carried out, for example, "letter sent," "referral to _____ made." But in the stream of behavior, it is not always easy to determine what responses by either the participant or the researcher are likely to contaminate the research. As we shall discuss later, interviews and other contacts with patient/subjects during the study should have as much realism as possible. In some cases, that means they will mimic clinical interactions. Always have notes recorded after every patient contact. These notes may suggest additional research contaminants later when you are reviewing them in your researcher role.

(4) *Collaborate* with one or more colleagues who have considerable research experience, preferably from outside the setting. If you cannot formally collaborate, at least have them read your proposal and/or talk with you about your research project. They may be able to foresee conflicts you cannot or provide creative solutions based on their past experience.

(5) *Separate yourself* from the role conflict. As a health professional, your clinical experience is probably more extensive than your research experience. Your most "natural" responses will arise from that clinical experience. If at all possible, use someone with more research than clinical experience to collect data and interact with the patient for the purposes of the research.

## CONSTRUCTING THE
## RESEARCH TEAM

Doing research in health care settings requires the expertise of both clinicians and researchers. Although there are "clinical researchers" and "research clinicians," it is, as discussed above, extremely difficult to combine successfully both roles in one person. The perspectives, goals, and trained responses are different. The single person trying to combine both roles will admit in all honesty that she or he either is really more one than the other or else is in a perpetual state of conflict. On the other hand, having the roles represented by different people can also lead to conflict—external, interpersonal conflict. Understanding and managing this conflict is one of the most challenging aspects of collaborative research.

## Finding the Right Expert

The team should be made up of people with knowledge of and experience with all the major substantive issues. There should be someone with expertise in the medical or health issues and the social or behavioral issues. There should be expert statistical consultation. If an unusual method of sampling is to be used, there should be someone who has experience with it. Someone familiar with the setting or patient care issues is valuable. Determining which experts are needed depends on the focus and complexity of the research project. Figure out your own "dream team" at the beginning. Then talk to possible members. Be as specific as possible about what the project needs from them. They may suggest the involvement of others for specific purposes.

It is extremely important to involve the needed experts *from the beginning*. Statistical consultants commonly complain that their advice is sought after the data are collected. Their input into the response format and coding scheme can result in a more flexible and useful data set. Similarly, a behavioral or social scientist should be consulted before any questionnaire is used to collect data. The wording and ordering of questions can make a huge difference in the quality of the data. A medical person should confirm that you are collecting the best health-status information possible.

## Defining Roles

In health care, physicians are usually at the top. They are accustomed to being able to give orders and assume authority, and other health professionals are also accustomed to this arrangement. There is a quite well-defined "pecking order." The outside researcher, whether brought in as a consultant or an initiator of research, has some difficulty finding an appropriate place in this hierarchy. Research credentials may not have the same weight in the health care setting as the academic setting, and there may be some initial posturing and jockeying for position among potential members of the research team. This is to be expected and is usual in the early stages of research. It is a disaster if it continues throughout the project.

An important first step in resolving this problem is to *define roles,* not as they are defined in the health or academic setting, but *in terms of the specific project.* Because you are constructing a team, it is likely that there are separable aspects of the project such as medical, social/behavioral, and statistical. Team members should know what their roles are and where their responsibilities fit into the project as a whole. A good rule is always to *put it in writing.* The role and responsibilities of each team member should be written out in as much detail as possible. These descriptions should also match reality as closely as possible and should be rewritten as that reality changes.

Another major problem in research projects involving a group is *ownership.* Someone had the original idea. Other people made it better. Some did more actual work than others. Someone provided access to resources. In general, contributions were made by more than one person, and the value of those contributions may be seen differently depending on where you stand. "Ownership" of the project may become blurred. In funded research, usually only one person is designated the Principal Investigator (PI), responsible for both the scientific and fiscal conduct of the research. Many institutions have requirements about who may serve as PI, for example, only a tenured faculty member, only a department head, only a dean. It may seem a trivial administrative detail that someone who is not the true "owner" of the project have this formal title, but it can lead to considerable conflict. The power of roles is such that assumption of the title for whatever reason is followed by increasing assumption of the role. Again, it is better to reflect reality in the job descriptions and titles or reality may change to reflect what is written. *Publication credit* is a related problem, which is also subject to formal rules of disciplines and institutions. Assigning publication credit will be discussed in more detail in Chapter 10. The important thing to note here is to *work it out in advance.*

## Working in a Team

Regular meetings are a good way for setting up an ongoing negotiation process for defining roles, clarifying communication, and resolving disputes. These meetings can be more or less formal depending on the size of the team. Sometimes formalizing roles like chair and recorder, which can either be fixed or rotate among team members, can facilitate the process. The objective is to maintain the agenda while allowing for problem resolution.

Problems can arise because people have different research styles and/or work habits. Some prefer early morning or late afternoon meetings. Some work best under pressure and leave everything to the last minute. Some can stand the delay of gratification involved in longitudinal research, and others need immediate results. More important than these style differences can be major conflicts about the quality of the final product. Research always requires a compromise between the ideal and the practical. The compromise can become a conflict between "getting it done" versus "doing it right." The quality judgments can be influenced by one's expertise and involvement in the project. Some people will simply care more, or they may care more about particular things that others think are trivial. Even defining "doing it right" can become a problem.

Involvement in the project and work styles also affect how team members spend their time. For some, this project will be the most important thing they are doing. They will be prepared to put aside other obligations and devote time to long, intense work periods. For others, it will be only one of several projects and commitments. Although they may be serious about their interest, the long-term consequences of the project may mean less in terms of their lives. Knowledge of the degree of commitment and the meaning of the project for each team member can minimize conflict over these differences. Focus should be maintained on the value of the substantive contributions of the team members.

## The Joys of Collaboration

Focusing on these problems of collaboration can obscure the very real benefits. An interdisciplinary team can be exciting and creative. Members bring fresh perspectives, new ideas and methods, and problem-solving as well as problem-generating capacities. It can be a substantive learning experience for all involved. Most important, it can produce a much better research product with more meaning and applicability for the health issue under study.

## SUMMARY

Health care settings are defined broadly to include not only physicians' offices but hospitals, clinics, nursing homes, voluntary health associations, the workplace, and other community settings. Health care is also defined broadly, and all medical personnel, including allied health professions, are considered health care professionals. Settings are reviewed in terms of their primary purpose, considerations affecting the population likely to be found there, and the impact on research of these features of the setting. "Outsider" issues are discussed in terms of a researcher outside the setting gaining and maintaining access for research purposes. Both formal and informal decision-making structures vary by setting and need to be identified. Strategies for obtaining physician cooperation are outlined. "Insider" issues are discussed in terms of role conflict, and strategies for minimizing these conflicts are suggested.

Constructing an interdisciplinary research team involves identifying the substantive issues and specific procedures of the project that require expertise. It is important to define roles and responsibilities clearly and in writing. Social and interpersonal conflicts that can arise because of differences in research styles and work habits are discussed. Finally, the joys and benefits of collaboration are mentioned.

## EXERCISES

(1) You wish to provide and evaluate a weight loss program that involves both diet and exercise. You can either recruit participants through the hospital in which you work (patients or employees) or use the patients of a private group medical practice or the employees of a local fast-food chain. How are these settings different in ways that might influence your study?

(2) Visit a local emergency room of a large hospital. How are the patients in the waiting room different from patients you might expect in the waiting room of a private group medical practice? What features of the setting have contributed to these differences?

# 3

## *Asking Research Questions*

Why do we do research? We do research because we are excited about a question and want to know the answer. Yet, defining the question and translating it into researchable terms can be one of the most intimidating parts of starting a research project. It can be intimidating to read the titles of research reports in journals. A title like "Attributions, Vulnerability, and Psychological Adjustment: The Case of Breast Cancer" (Timko & Janoff-Bulman, 1985) may have started as a question like "Do you think that people's judgments about the causes of their diseases affect coping?" or "What if we asked breast cancer patients why they think they have breast cancer?" A formal title is the final expression of a research question that started out as a good idea.

Ideas come from many sources, but the evaluation of the essential goodness of the idea starts with you. How do you know if you have a good idea? A good idea is one you personally love. If you are excited about it, you will discuss it in informal settings, with colleagues, friends, and family. You will then have an opportunity to clarify it and to be able to express it to many possible audiences. You will have gotten valuable feedback. It is also important to love your idea because you have to live with most research projects for a long time, from conception to final research report. If you are only lukewarm now, you will hate it by the end, or, worse yet, you may never finish it!

A good idea is also one that someone else may be interested in, one that has implications outside your immediate circle or the research team. Can you imagine yourself on the Phil Donohue show talking about your research? Can you express it clearly for that type of audience and make it interesting to them? Would they care? Maybe not. Sometimes you have to strain to think who else might be interested. It is worth going through that exercise at the beginning of the research to provide some perspective.

A good idea need not start out as your own. The major research question may have been developed by someone else and you are approached to participate on the research team. It is important at this point to examine the proposed project carefully to see whether there is a particular piece of it you can get excited about. You should, of course, have an overall positive reaction to the proposal before you commit yourself to the project, but the point here is to make some small part of it your own, to add your perspective and the value of your experiences, to care about some part of the outcome personally, and to see that piece through from beginning to end. In the very earliest stages of your career, it may be helpful to participate in a research team solely to get experience without thinking that you have to make a major, substantive contribution. Even in this case, however, it is probably better to care about some aspect of the research.

## APPROACHES TO
## HEALTH ISSUES

Medical professionals and behavioral scientists may take quite different approaches to questions relating to health. And even within these fields, there are often different approaches depending on background and training.

### Medical Approaches

One medical approach typically defines the problem beginning with the disease entity, such as cancer, arthritis, heart or lung conditions. A second medical approach (also identified with public health) focuses on the stage of health care, such as prevention, early detection and screening, recovery, or rehabilitation and adaptation to chronic illness. This approach recognizes that there may be issues at each of these stages that cut across diseases. A third approach might focus on the nature of the treatment needed such as surgery or medication/chemotherapy. Thus someone could be interested in cancer and in what factors are related to onset of the disease, its progress, or its remission. Another person might focus on early cancer detection or rehabilitation issues. A third might focus on responses to chemotherapy. The nature of their questions and hypotheses would be very different.

### Psychological or Behavioral Approaches

Psychological or behavioral approaches are concerned with people's responses to health and illness. The focus might be on compliance, perceived control over health outcomes, the relation between attitudes and preventive behavior, or responses to stressors. Two different perspectives are taken on these issues. One focuses on the individual or aspects of the person. The other focuses on the aspects of the setting or situation. Thus an individual focus might lead to questions about which cancer patients adapt well to the disease or engage in early detection or comply with their regimens. A situational focus might lead to questions about how others respond to cancer patients in ways that affect their adaptation, or how the nature of the medication regimen or side effects enhance compliance.

## Choosing the Focus

Clearly, health research questions can have more than one focus. Selecting the major focus when any or all of these may be appropriate is a problem for the researcher. To provide another example, one could be interested in breast self-examination from a number of directions. Medically, the question might be the efficacy of BSE in detecting small tumors or cancer at an early stage of the disease. Put in the context of early detection, the use of breast self-examination might be compared to mammography or even blood pressure screening. An individually oriented psychologist might be interested in which people comply with BSE, while a psychologist with a situational focus might look at enhancing environmental cues to increase compliance, as we did (Grady, 1984). Research projects can be designed to shed some light on all of these issues, but the primary focus must be selected.

It makes sense to have a primary focus (medical or psychological) especially as difficult decisions become necessary and trade-offs must be made in planning the research. Much research in health care settings, however, combines more than one of these foci. It is when some aspect of the design needs to be cut, some measures eliminated, and other such decisions made that a primary focus is most critical. How do you choose the focus and sort out its priority? There are several general considerations you should take into account.

*(1) Start with yourself.* What is your personal interest? As we said above, the research should engage you. The focus should also reflect your training and background. It makes sense to deal from strength. Psychologists who focus on disease and physicians who specialize in attitudes are outside their major areas of expertise and often do not make the contribution they could. Your personal strengths and

weaknesses are also important. Some people can be comfortable around critically ill patients while others are not. Some people are particularly successful in dealing with children while others are not. Longitudinal research can provide rich opportunities for some and delay gratification beyond endurance for others. You need to assess your personal style and abilities realistically when selecting a research focus.

*(2) Evaluate the research team.* The research team is also critical in selecting a focus. What areas of expertise, interest, and personal strengths are represented on the team? What additional resource people can be brought in to supplement them? Who can you call on for occasional advice or feedback about the idea? With what literature are the team members familiar to ensure that the idea is current? The nature of the question determines who is needed on the team, but the composition of the team also shapes the nature of the question.

*(3) Consider available funding.* If you want funding, you need to be aware of the nature of granting agencies. For example, in the federal government, most agencies are organized by disease. If your interest is compliance, it will be easier to obtain funding for a question on compliance related to a specific disease, such as hypertension, than for studies that go across disease entities. In the control studies described in Example 3.1, we continually had to justify to our funding agency research that cut across diseases.

*(4) Consider the intended audience.* Questions with a solely psychological focus may be of interest to you and your psychology colleagues but physicians may say "so what?" If your goal is policy change, you must consider the nature of the policymaking audience and the kinds of questions that will be relevant. Journal outlets that you are most likely to choose or conventions at which presentations will be made also suggest what concerns your audience/readers are likely to have.

---

*Example 3.1.*
*Choosing the Focus*

Three psychologists wanted to do theory-based field experiments in health care settings. One of us had a background as a nurse, which probably contributed to our decision about the setting. All three of us had personal styles that involved desiring control over our lives. We also shared humanitarian values about patients' rights to choose their health care treatments. We therefore decided that the major research focus would be on patient control through treatment choices. Our background and training as social psychologists led us to investigate both individual characteristics and situational factors that might be related to exercising this control.

We realized that we needed additional medical knowledge in order to select treatments where choice would be possible. We found a physician to join our team. He suggested that patients could have choices about the manner of preparation for barium enema X-rays. We also found another investigator who was already involved in research on different treatments for emesis (vomiting) from cancer chemotherapy. Collaborating with him also provided knowledge of chemotherapy, setting entry, and assistance with measures by coordinating our work with his. We added a nurse researcher with medical/surgical background to facilitate study design and conduct. Thus we developed collaborative studies on patients' choice of treatment for two different medical procedures. It was the interests of the original team members, however, that most affected our continuing focus as trade-offs became necessary in the study design.

---

## GENERATING RESEARCH IDEAS

Just as the formal title of a research article may be quite different from the question, or idea, the introduction that reviews the literature does not really tell us the source of the idea. We are taught to couch our studies in terms of previous research and theory. While this is sometimes where we get our research ideas, there are countless other sources possible. (See McGuire, 1983, for a more thorough discussion of some of these.) We elaborate just a few.

(1) One really good source is *observing the real world*. Science, after all, starts with systematic observation. If you are a health professional, you have much experience from which to generate research questions. You may have noticed for some time that patients who don't ask a lot of questions take a lot longer to recover from surgery or suffer more anxiety. This kind of observation or informal "hunch" is the stuff of which research questions are made. If you are not a health care professional, it might be helpful to do some observation in a health care setting that is of interest.

(2) You can also use *your own experience*. Imagining yourself as a participant in your study or a member of the target group can be critically valuable in framing your question, choosing what you will actually do and what you will measure. (See Example 3.2.) Role-playing being a patient going through a procedure (where possible) can provide

some insights into the patient perspective for health care practitioners and other researchers.

---

*Example 3.2.*
*Personal Observation/Experience*

I had spent countless hours in the library, reading the literature on women's practice of breast self-examination (BSE). The articles consisted of some research studies, some editorials in major medical journals, and some essays. The research base was very weak, mainly surveys asking some group of women whether they did BSE, and, if not, why not. The groups often were not large or representative. The questions and format varied tremendously from study to study. That most women did not do it was clear, having been found repeatedly. Why they did not do it was not at all clear. I was developing a long list of possible reasons women did not do it. They seemed to fall into three categories: (1) women were ignorant of how or why to do BSE; (2) women were too modest to touch themselves; and (3) women were too fearful of what they would find. The reasons all seemed quite plausible, but somehow were not satisfactory. The question kept repeating itself, "Why *don't* women do BSE?" Then I asked the question of myself, "Why don't I do BSE?" I knew none of the reasons explained my behavior. Then I changed the question: "What would get me to do it?" It occurred to me that, if a friend called each month and asked if I had done it, I would do it, either in anticipation of her call or immediately afterward. Changing the question to a positive one completely changed my way of thinking about the problem: "What would *encourage* women to do BSE?" The new question opened a range of possibilities by putting BSE in the context of behavior modification, which offered a variety of testable techniques for changing behavior.

---

(3) *Interviewing patients* also will increase your understanding of situations and generate ideas. *Intensive case studies* are a form of personal experience/systematic observation, which is a good source of questions. Health care professionals can easily incorporate such case studies into their day-to-day activities.

(4) *General reading* can also provide insight for hypotheses. Biographies, autobiographies, and novels that concern health care issues provide a way of observing the world. Norman Cousins's (1979) book *Anatomy of an Illness* provides a perspective on the health care system and aspects of patient recovery worth studying.

(5) *Practitioner's rules of thumb,* the things you may do without knowing why, may be an excellent source of hypotheses. Many of these

develop from experience and when examined further are hypotheses worth testing. Many practitioners believe that talking to patients in a coma improves their chances of recovery. Systematic research testing this idea could help us determine whether it is worth the obviously high cost in staff time.

(6) *Examining an opposite problem* can be an interesting approach. For example, lack of compliance with drug regimens involves underuse of drugs and substance abuse involves overuse. Anorexia involves undereating and obesity involves overeating. It may be possible to suggest reciprocal solutions to the problems by contrasting the factors involved (McGuire, 1983).

(7) There are a series of more traditional question generating sources. In the *hypothetico-deductive method,* you begin with a theory and use logical deductions to derive a set of predictions. For example, learned helplessness is a theory that explains people's responses to severe negative events that are not under their control. In general, it has been found that people get depressed and apathetic. We recognize that some chronic illnesses might fit the pattern and are currently studying persons with rheumatoid arthritis to see the extent to which learned helplessness develops.

(8) In addition to theory, previous data are a source of questions. When two studies have *conflicting results,* coming up with some way to explain them produces a new hypothesis. We had found that people who believed that they were responsible for their own health and who valued their health sought more information about hypertension (Wallston, Maides, & Wallston, 1976). We tried to replicate the study using a slightly different scale several years later and did not get this finding. We realized that there had been much press coverage of hypertension, so we hypothesized that the difference between the studies had to do with novelty of the information at the time of the first study. We therefore planned a study that included hypertension and a more novel disease (at that time), herpes. The journal *Disease-A-Month* was helpful in choosing a disease. We predicted that we would get the finding for herpes and not for hypertension information-seeking. Unfortunately, our prediction did not work. In fact, we got the expected results for hypertension and not herpes. We have not yet come up with an explanation, and, for the time being, this research is in a file drawer.

(9) Similar to conflicting findings are *exceptions to general findings* as a hypothesis source. If you can figure out why the exception occurs, you have a new hypothesis to test.

(10) *Observed complex relationships* can be categorized into simpler components. The process of preparation for surgery has generated much research with studies generally showing that information provided before the surgery is related to better outcomes afterward. Johnson and Leventhal (1974) suggested that the type of information might be even more strongly related to outcomes with a noxious medical procedure (endoscopy). They distinguished behavioral information from information on sensations or what the patient can expect to feel. It was found that a combination of these types of information was most successful for reducing distress and increasing patient compliance.

(11) Conceptual analyses also provide a source of ideas. *Analogy* is a creative and uncommon approach to hypothesis generation. It involves transferring concepts from one arena to another. For example, McGuire (1973) borrowed the term "inoculation" from medicine to describe a method of developing resistance to attitude change. *Reversing the direction* of a commonsense hypothesis can encourage one to think of the conditions under which it would hold. For example, it seems to make sense that people want to feel in control. But Wortman reversed this relationship and suggested that feeling in control when one gets cancer might lead to self-blame and use of quack treatments (Wortman & Dunkle-Schetter, 1979). Similarly, the focus or direction between independent and dependent variables can be reversed. We started our arthritis study expecting severe disease to increase patients' sense of helplessness. Instead, we found that increased helplessness seemed to increase severity or functional disability.

(12) *Policy* is a particularly rich source of health research questions. The general term *policy* covers decision making at many levels. Policy issues can range from local decisions in a hospital, such as whether to use primary nursing (where a nurse has ongoing responsibility for specific patients) or to rotate assignments, to current state legislative controversies over mandatory seat-belt laws, to congressional action related to Medicaid reimbursement. Such policy issues can provide inspiration for research, and research can provide useful information. Many policy decisions are based on scant research findings rather than cost considerations. Health policy is often made from the viewpoint of administrators, and additional research that explicates effects on other parts of the system, including patients, can be valuable.

For example, Senator William S. Cohen (1985) of Maine in an *American Psychologist* forum discusses the value of health promotion in the workplace. He discusses a number of different programs, including stress management. Turning his assertions into policy-related hypotheses, one could test whether stress management programs in the workplace decrease absenteeism or health insurance cost and increase productivity. Based on belief in the value of such programs (enhanced by research), Cohen has introduced the Preventive Health Care Incentive Act, providing a tax credit to employers who provide such programs for employees.

## REFINING THE QUESTION

Not all interesting questions make good research questions. A research question must be relatively narrow and feasible. Above all, a research question must be a genuine question in that the answers obtained can support or fail to support the hypothesis. A question such as "Does stress cause cancer?" is certainly interesting but a single research project cannot answer it. Stress is also a very broad concept. One would have to think through more precisely what one means by "stress" and then decide how to go about measuring it. In research terms, stress is the *construct* or general concept you are interested in and the specific measures are attempts to *operationalize* that construct.

Feasibility is a major issue in health research. People cannot be randomly assigned a health status. Many diseases and conditions are relatively rare. Many things we want to know about, such as psychological status, cannot be directly observed. There are large intuitive leaps from physiological measures to psychological and physical impact, especially long-term effects. These issues will be discussed further in the chapters on design, measurement, and interpretation. As a study is designed and specific procedures and measures are chosen, the research question will become increasingly refined.

### The Basic Elements

A good research question has at least three major elements: two variables and a relationship between them. A *variable* must have two or more different levels or values. For example, compliance with a medical regimen is a variable in that people can be more or less compliant. It can be measured as levels: using only two levels, people's behavior could be classified as compliant or not compliant; using three levels, the classifications could be very compliant, somewhat compliant, or not compliant; using multiple levels, the behavior could be measured in terms of how many pills are taken in a given time. If the research question concerned the relationship between severity of illness and compliance, severity of illness must also be conceptualized as a variable that could take on two or more values. If the research question concerned an intervention to increase compliance, that intervention must also have a minimum of two levels (presence/absence).

The presumed nature of the relationship between the variables determines what they are called. If the relationship is presumed to be causal, the variable thought to cause changes or differences is labeled the *independent variable*. The independent variable must be under the control of the researcher and independent of what the study participant does. In the compliance example, the intervention would be an independent variable. The variable that is hypothesized to change as a result of the intervention is the *dependent variable* in that the resulting values will depend on the intervention. In the compliance example, the dependent variable would be the measure of compliance. Other variables on which study participants may differ and that might affect the dependent variable can be treated as *control variables*. Their presumed relationship is important enough to be identified and measured, but the researcher wishes to minimize their effects in order to obtain a clearer test of the hypothesis. In the compliance example, severity of illness could be treated as a control variable by separating participants into groups depending on their severity of illness and then testing the effects of the intervention within each of these groups.

## Searching the Literature

When you have a general idea about your question, as part of the task of refining it, you need to find out what other people have asked and found out relevant to your question. This search of the literature used to take countless hours in the library, but the computer era has speeded up the process. There are several major computer information services that can be accessed through your library (or your home computer if you join a telecommunications network like Dialog, Source, or CompuServe). These services abstract most of the journals of interest to you. PsychInfo provides primary access to the psychology literature. Medline includes most of the medical literature. What you will get from computer searches of these sources depends very much on the *key words* you select. Reference librarians can be very helpful in assisting your selection. You should search for key words that are related to the variables in your question, the specific measures you have chosen, and the diseases or health areas you are studying. For other details on conducting literature searches, see Cooper (1984).

## Stating the Hypothesis

We can go a step beyond our question and assert our hunch in the form of a hypothesis. Usually, when we have a question, we have some guess as to its answer. We then assert or hypothesize the expected relationship between the variables. Although, in statistics class, you may have been pushed to specify null hypotheses or the assertion of no difference between the groups, a directional hypothesis should be specified when suggested by theory, observation, or previous research.

Drawing a picture of the presumed relationship between the variables can help clarify your hypothesis. Imagine the results you would obtain should your hunch be correct. In the compliance example, you might expect an overall positive correlation (relationship) between severity of illness and compliance, that is, the sicker one is, the more compliant with the medication. Graphing this hypothesized relationship might raise additional questions: Is it true that you expect increased compliance for every level of illness? Perhaps it is only among the very ill that the relationship will hold. Graphing alternative hypotheses and evaluating their plausibility may help you refine your question further.

## SUMMARY

We do research because we have a question we want to answer. Questions in health care can be from a medical/public health or a psychological/behavioral perspective. Most interdisciplinary research involves both. Choosing a primary focus is particularly important to guide difficult decisions about the design of the study and trade-offs during its conduct. Four general considerations are given for choosing the focus: yourself, the research team, the funding source, and the intended audience. Research ideas can be generated from a variety of sources other than the traditional reliance on past research and theory. Starting with observing the real world and your own experience, 12 sources of ideas for questions are given. To refine the question, three basic elements must be identified: two variables and a relationship between them. A directional hypothesis about the relationship should be stated if at all possible.

## EXERCISES

(1) Devise a research question based on each of the following ideas mentioned in this chapter: the benefits of talking to people in comas; the use of quack treatments by people with cancer; similarities between undereating (anorexia) and overeating (obesity); the effectiveness of mandatory seat-belt laws; primary care nursing. Refine each question so that the three major elements are clear. If possible, state the question in the form of a specific hypothesis.

(2) Select key words to conduct a literature search relevant to two of the hypotheses generated above.

# 4

## *Designing the Study*

The research design specifies the number of groups in a study, when the interventions (if any) will occur, and, most important, the order and frequency of observations or measures. By the time you finalize your design, you will have given considerable thought to the purposes of the research, what information is needed, what data are feasible and not feasible to collect, who the study participants will be, and many other aspects of the study. It is also important, however, to give early consideration to what general type of design is appropriate for your research question.

There are three general types of designs, each of which will be discussed in this chapter. All of the designs have strengths and weaknesses, and an evaluation of their features should be part of the initial study planning. There are three general questions that discriminate among the major types of design:

(1) Is there a planned treatment or intervention?
(2) Will there be a control group comparison?
(3) Is random assignment to groups possible?

If there is no planned treatment or intervention, but rather you are planning to survey or to monitor a sample over time, the design is a *correlational* one. If there will be a control group comparison but random assignment to groups is not possible, the design is a *quasi-experimental* one. If there is only one subject or object of a study (a single patient, one hospital, one state), the design is also quasi-experimental. If there will be one or more control groups in the study and random assignment of participants to treatment and control groups, the design is *experimental.*

Designs in health research are often mixed. For example, in an experimental design, questionnaire or interview data will often be collected before or after the intervention from both the experimental and the control group. These data can then be used correlationally to describe the relationship among variables that characterize the sample. In addition, the sample can be divided into groups based on a response to one of the interview questions, and differences between these groups can be examined. This approach would be quasi-experimental in that there was no random assignment to groups but rather the groups were created on the basis of a response.

Designs may also be used sequentially to answer a research question in a series of studies. If one wishes to increase medication compliance, but had very little idea of the factors that might be affecting it, one could start with a correlational study, interviewing people who vary in compliance and who vary on some factors that are candidates for intervention. For example, one might want to know about the medication regimen itself (frequency, amount, side effects) or health-status variables, social situation, or personality factors of the patients. This study would be *exploratory* and possibly hypothesis-generating for subsequent experimental or quasi-experimental studies. In the follow-up experimental study, the factor presumed to cause the compliance could be systematically varied to provide a stronger test of its effects.

Another sequence of studies might proceed from experimental to correlational designs. One might wish to test whether effects demonstrated under tightly controlled experimental conditions are evident under less controlled, more naturalistic conditions. For example, there is a large body of "learned helplessness" literature, which demonstrates that unavoidable aversive events lead to giving up or lack of trying to avoid them (Seligman, 1975). This demonstrated laboratory relationship is now being tested by us in a correlational study of people with rheumatoid arthritis to determine whether uncontrollable flares of the disease lead to a sense of helplessness and decreased everyday functioning.

## Validity

The major concern in experimental designs and the basis on which they are judged as strong or weak is validity. Validity determines the extent to which we may have confidence in the soundness of our conclusions. Threats to validity provide alternative explanations for the observed results. There are two major kinds of validity. *Internal validity* refers to the truth of the statement that A caused B in a specific study. Threats to internal validity offer *rival hypotheses,* mostly in the form of something else being just as likely to have caused B. *External validity* refers to whether the relationship between variables found in the particular study will be found elsewhere with different populations, settings, treatments, and measures. In this chapter, designs will be evaluated primarily for internal validity. External validity or *generalizability* will be discussed further in Chapter 5, on sample selection, and in

Chapter 10, on inference. (See Cook & Campbell, 1979; and Huck & Sandler, 1979, for more extensive discussions of validity issues.)

Different designs control for different threats to validity. No design is perfect, as we discussed in Chapter 1; each presents different dilemmas of interpretation that must be taken into account. This chapter does not attempt to describe all possible designs but rather to give an overview of some of the strengths and weaknesses of some major designs that are applied in health research. The reader is referred to other design books for elaboration. We shall begin with correlational designs, then describe some common designs that Campbell and Stanley (1963) label as "preexperimental designs" in order to demonstrate the weaknesses that experimental designs are intended to overcome. Finally, we shall cover quasi-experimental and experimental designs.

## CORRELATIONAL DESIGNS

Correlational designs are nonexperimental designs in that there is no intervention or treatment. They involve collecting data on two or more variables and exploring the relationship between them. A major advantage of correlational designs is the ability to investigate complex relationships between many variables in a single study. Several competing hypotheses about the relationships between and among variables can be tested at once. If two variables measured do not significantly covary, that is, if the correlation is near zero, the hypothesis that there is a relationship between them can be judged unlikely to be true. If they do covary, then there is a relationship between them and there are grounds for future studies. Subsequent experimental studies could test causality and the conditions under which the relationship holds.

A major disadvantage to correlational designs is that causality cannot be assumed from demonstrated relationships. For example, height and breast cancer rates appear to be related, but it is highly unlikely that either one causes the other (Micozzi, 1985). The terms *predictors* and *criteria* are used rather than independent and dependent variables to emphasize the point. Which variable is the independent variable or predictor and which is the dependent variable or criterion is relatively arbitrary. Nonetheless, correlational designs are sometimes the only choice available and can provide valuable data. If such findings can be replicated and supplemented by other kinds of data, a convincing *argument* for causality can be made. All the data supporting the smoking/lung-cancer relationship, for example, are based on correlational studies, and taken together, are quite convincing that smoking causes lung cancer. To make a logical argument that there is a causal relationship between variables in a correlational study, three conditions must be met: (1) the predictors and criterion must covary, (2) the predictors must precede the criterion in time, and (3) there must be no good alternative explanations of the relationship.

### Cross-Sectional (Single-Shot) Designs

This is the weakest and the most frequent correlational design. All variables are measured at a single point in time, using, for example, a questionnaire or interview administered to some group. There are many potential alternative explanations for why relationships among variables may be observed. Variables that are measured at a single point in time tend to be related more than those measured at different points. This similarity may be because study participants are responding to the same interviewer, in the same setting, in the same mood, or striving for consistency in reports of behavior, attitudes, and health status. Other biases in self-report, which will be discussed in Chapter 7, may enter into the responses. Furthermore, either variable may cause the other or they may both be caused by a third variable that may or may not have been measured in the study. Example 4.1 describes an attempt to argue causality from correlational data.

---

*Example 4.1.*
*Which Came First?*

In a cross-sectional design, we surveyed persons with epilepsy (DeVellis, DeVellis, Wallston, & Wallston, 1980). Based on learned helplessness theory (Seligman, 1975), we hypothesized that the more one's epilepsy history was characterized by unpredictable and uncontrollable seizures, the more helpless one would feel. We operationalized helplessness as depression and certain locus of control beliefs. We found that epilepsy history did relate to helplessness so we satisfied condition one (covariation) of the three conditions for arguing causality. We tried to argue that the epilepsy history variable logically preceded helplessness, although we measured all of the variables at the same time. We have no real way of knowing people's beliefs or level of depression *before* the onset of epilepsy, however, and, therefore, the requirement that the predictors must precede the criterion in time is not satisfied. Moreover, because some of our epilepsy history variables required subjective judgments (e.g., the predictability and controllability of seizures), it is plausible to argue that depression or beliefs about health might cause people to describe their seizures differently. Thus there are alternative plausible explanations of our conclusions.

---

Sometimes cross-sectional designs are used to approximate the effects of time or aging by comparing different groups. It is important to recognize in such cases that, at best, we can talk about differences between groups. We cannot conclude anything about increases or decreases. We have shown, for example, that people who are older tend to desire less control over their health care than do younger people (Woodward & Wallston, 1986). While we tried to make a logical case that aging leads to or causes a decrease in such beliefs, this is not a clear conclusion from such cross-sectional data. In other words, the particular experiences of these age groupings may be different, and such differences would not always develop as part of the aging process. The difference would then be the result of a *cohort effect* rather than an *age effect*. Cohort effects are always possible alternative explanations for correlational age effects. Will these younger people decrease in desire for control as they age? Only by following the sample over time (a *longitudinal* design) can conclusions about increases or decreases with age be reached.

## Longitudinal Designs

In a longitudinal design, data are collected at more than one point in time. These are relatively costly and are, therefore, not as common in health care research studies as they are in discussion sections setting out what should be done (Kobasa, 1985). Longitudinal designs can establish the temporal (time) relationship between variables, that is, which variable precedes and predicts which other variable. Example 4.2 illustrates a longitudinal design with an unexpected finding. It should be noted that, even with temporal precedence established, the causal direction of the relationship still requires a logical argument.

---

*Example 4.2.*
*An Unexpected Finding*

We are continuing our interest in learned helplessness as it relates to chronic illness through a longitudinal study of persons with rheumatoid arthritis (RA). Questionnaires are administered every six months to a sample of RA patients over a three-and-one-half-year period. As with the epilepsy study (Example 4.1), the hypothesis is that disease severity will lead to increased helplessness. By measuring both arthritis severity and helplessness at each of the six-month intervals, this temporal relationship can be tested.

The initial results for the first two time periods produced an interesting and unexpected finding. Contrary to the hypothesis, arthritis severity at time 1 did not predict helplessness at time 2. Helplessness at time 1 did, however, predict severity at time 2. After the fact, this finding makes a great deal of sense. Severity was measured in terms of pain and functional ability. Helplessness may lead to decreased attempts at activity when there is pain, and this would show up as increased severity, with people reporting that they can do less and less without help. At time 1 and at time 2, helplessness and severity are correlated. Thus if we had done only the cross-sectional analysis, we would have concluded incorrectly that severity leads to helplessness. Clearly, much more information about the potential for causation is available from longitudinal data. In terms of the three requirements for causation, cross-sectional designs allow us only to assure covariation between predictors and criteria. Longitudinal designs allow us to assess that predictors precede the criterion in time. The third requirement, of no good alternative explanation of a relationship, always requires a logical argument.

## Prospective Designs

A prospective design provides the strongest potential for causal conclusions of the correlational designs. The predictors are measured *prior to* the criterion, a major requirement for causal conclusion. Prospective designs are difficult and costly, however, when studying unpredictable, infrequent events. Consider the learned helplessness studies. It would take an incredibly large sample at the outset to measure beliefs and depression *before* the onset of chronic illness. If rheumatoid arthritis affects 1 in 100 40-year-olds, a sample of at least 10,000 people younger than 40 would be necessary to expect to obtain a sample of 100 study participants who would get RA at age 40. Such a costly venture would not be warranted without strong evidence in favor of the hypothesis. More frequent criterion events are needed for feasible prospective studies.

## TWO EXAMPLES OF
## PROBLEMATIC DESIGNS

The following designs are offered as problematic examples of scientific research. Each of them has major weaknesses in terms of internal validity—the ability to infer causation. They provide an opportunity to describe the nature of these threats to validity, as Campbell and Stanley (1963) used them in their classic book on experimental and quasi-experimental designs. We do not mean to say that they are never appropriate, and sometimes they are the best that can be done under given circumstances. Many times, however, they can be improved substantially by adding some of the controls or multiple instances of measurement that will be described later in the chapter.

## One-Group Pretest Posttest

In this common treatment design, an observation or measurement is taken before an intervention and repeated afterward. Using "O" to indicate observation and "X" for treatment or intervention, the design can be illustrated as follows:

$$O_1 \times O_2$$

Although any changes observed might at first glance appear attributable to X, in fact, there are numerous other plausible rival hypotheses or reasons why O at time 2 could have changed from that at time 1. We shall describe five such threats to validity. (1) Something other than the treatment/intervention may have occurred between the two observations that could account for a change in O, a rival hypothesis referred to as *history*. The longer the time lag between the two observations, the stronger this possibility. (2) The study participants themselves may have changed between the two observations in some biological or psychological way that would normally change over time, a threat called *maturation*. This kind of change is one that has nothing to do with the study but could possibly affect the measure of outcomes.

There are also changes that could result because of the study itself. (3) Simply taking a test twice can result in changes in scores because of increasing familiarity with or understanding of the responses that are desirable; this *testing* alternative hypothesis is equally valid for any kind of measure administered twice to the same sample. (4) If one uses slightly different measures the second time, then any changes observed could be due to *instrumentation*. Even without changes in the measures, there can be changes in how they are administered: interviewers can become more familiar with the instruments and provide more detailed data; observers can become more or less alert recording observations over time.

(5) There can also be changes because of *statistical regression,* which

involves changes in scores because measurement instruments themselves are unreliable and extreme scores tend to regress toward the mean. This alternative explanation is particularly plausible when study participants have been selected for very high or very low scores; they will tend to score closer to the mean when tested again. For example, if a screening and intervention program selected persons with high blood pressure readings, then provided a dietary intervention, the subsequent scores could be lower because of regression to the mean, which would be an alternative to the explanation that the dietary intervention itself improved blood pressure.

### Static Group Comparison

In this design, a control group is added for comparison to a group that has experienced some X. It should be noted that the researcher did not administer or control X nor randomly assign subjects/participants to groups. An example would be attempting to study the effects of existing groups such as Weight Watchers by comparing their weight loss to some other group. The design can be diagrammed as follows with the line indicating that there was no random assignment to groups:

$$\frac{X \; 0_1}{0_2}$$

There are two major threats to internal validity in this design. *Selection* refers to differences between people in the treatment and control groups. Selecting a control group that did not differ in some systematic way from the people in Weight Watchers would be difficult. Weight Watchers may be an effective treatment but issues such as the motivation of people who enroll can nearly always serve as a good alternative explanation. Another threat is *mortality,* that is, a loss of participants that is differential between the treatment and control group. It may be that the people who were not losing weight dropped out of Weight Watchers, leaving only the successful to be compared with the control group.

### QUASI-EXPERIMENTAL DESIGNS

Quasi-experimental designs represent efforts to control for many of the threats to internal validity described in the preexperimental designs.

A randomized experimental design, examples of which will be given in the next section, is always preferred as a way to infer causality. There are many times, however, particularly in health care research, when the researcher cannot control who receives the intervention and, therefore, cannot randomly assign participants to experimental and treatment conditions. By selecting appropriate control groups or by taking multiple measurements over time, the quasi-experimental design increases confidence in the test of whether the intervention or treatment caused a change in the outcome measured. There are many types of quasi-experiments, and more extensive coverage of them can be found in Campbell and Stanley (1963) and Cook and Campbell (1979).

## Nonequivalent Control Groups

The most common type of quasi-experiment is a nonequivalent control group design with pretest and posttest. Here a naturally occurring phenomenon, or one you can create, serves as the treatment. A similar group serves as the contrast or control group. (See Chapter 5 for information on control group selection.)

$$\frac{O_1 \times O_3}{O_2 \quad O_4}$$

For many threats to internal validity, having a control group and a premeasure can rule out many alternative explanations. To the extent that the control group experiences the same history, maturation, testing, instrumentation, and extremity of scores on the premeasure, then effects of these factors on the outcome measure would be reflected in changes in the control group as well as in the experimental group. Additional differences between the control group and the experimental group could then be said to have been caused by the treatment rather than these alternative factors. Two major threats to validity, however, remain: selection and mortality.

The term *nonequivalent* control group reminds us that, without random assignment, we cannot be certain that the two groups are equivalent. Group members may have either been selected differentially or have dropped out of the group differentially. The pretest attempts to confirm that there is equivalency between the groups on the measures of interest. It should be noted that the addition of even a nonequivalent control group in this design makes it far superior to the one-group pretest-posttest design discussed earlier. The more similar the method of recruitment and the scores on the pretest between the experimental and control groups, the stronger the control for selection and mortality.

## Multiple Control Groups/Posttest Only

Although pretests are very important, there are times when, for ethical or practical reasons, they are not possible. Example 4.3 describes an instance where an uncontrolled event was likely to have an impact on health, and the researchers for obvious reasons were unable to obtain a measure before the event. They chose multiple control groups for comparisons:

$$\times \quad \underline{\phantom{xx} 0_1 \phantom{xx}}$$

$$\underline{\phantom{xx} 0_2 \phantom{xx}}$$

$$\underline{\phantom{xx} 0_3 \phantom{xx}}$$

$$\underline{\phantom{xx} 0_4 \phantom{xx}}$$

Because all four groups are being tested at the same time, issues such as history, maturation, testing, instrumentation, and statistical regression do not apply. The major threats to validity in this design, as with all nonequivalent control group designs, are *selection* and *mortality*. The researchers specifically chose groups to test various selection hypotheses. They also collected information about study participants' backgrounds and characteristics (sociodemographics) to identify possible group differences. Given the nature of the question and the inherent limitations, this design presents an attempt to deal directly with the major threats to internal validity.

---

*Example 4.3.*
*Controlling for Selection Bias*

Baum, Gatchel, and Schaeffer (1983) wanted to evaluate the impact of a powerful environmental stressor, the nuclear accident at Three Mile Island (TMI), on mental health. Obviously, no pretest was possible. Obviously also, for ethical reasons, a powerful stressor such as this could never be studied using random assignment. To control for selection and environmental issues, Baum et al. chose three comparison groups: people living (a) near an undamaged nuclear plant, (b) near a coal-fired power plant, and (c) in an area more than 20 miles from any power plant. Selection would suggest that perhaps people who chose to live near TMI would have scored differently on the measures even without the stress of the near meltdown. The first comparison group then is another group of people who chose to live near a nuclear power plant. The second comparison group controls for living near a power plant of any type. The third comparison group tests the selection hypothesis by providing a sample that does not live near a power plant of any type. Areas sampled were comparable in socioeconomic status and were all in the northeast United States.

Using a series of self-report, performance, and physiological measures, it was found that, almost one and one-half years after the nuclear accident at TMI, residents reported more physical symptoms, anxiety, depression, and alienation; they performed worse on tasks requiring concentration; they also had higher sympathetic arousal. The three control groups did not differ. To rule out other selection factors, differences between groups were tested on background variables such as age, marital status, sex, education, and income. These variables were not related to outcome variables, and the lack of relationship implies that they cannot explain the findings. In a quasi-experiment, it is important to make as good a case as you can that the treatment and not other factors caused the difference between groups.

## Time Series

In a time-series design, multiple measures or observations are taken both before and after an intervention or treatment is introduced. A basic time-series design may be diagrammed as follows:

$$O_1 \; O_2 \; O_3 \; O_4 \times O_5 \; O_6 \; O_7 \; O_8$$

Time-series designs, which are much more common in the physical sciences, present a vast improvement over the pre-post design involving only a single measurement at each point as was described earlier. Because of the multiple measurements, many of the threats to internal validity can be ruled out as implausible rival hypotheses. History provides the strongest challenge because some other event could happen coincidentally with the intervention or treatment. Even weather changes or seasonal variations could contribute to a change because time series by nature happen over time. Such extraneous factors could account for any changes observed, a possibility that cannot be ruled out by this design and must be evaluated depending on the specific circumstances, topic, and measurement. Maturation, testing, instrumentation, and regression present very unlikely rival hypotheses because any effects they might have should be evident at various points in the measurement and are unlikely to happen only at the same time as the intervention. Selection and mortality effects do not apply as long as the same people or events are being measured at each point. In this sense, participants serve as their own controls.

The classic example of an interrupted time-series design involves an analysis of Connecticut's 1955 crackdown on speeding (Campbell, 1969). There was a year of record high fatalities followed by an extremely severe crackdown. When there was a 12.3% reduction in fatalities in the year of the crackdown, the program was seen as a success by policymakers and the public. When the decrease was put in the context of several years preceding and following the crackdown, its success could be more thoroughly evaluated. Because the year before the crackdown was a particularly high year, some *regression to the mean* would be expected. Having the perspective of a number of data points showed that the drop to fewer accidents was in fact not very different than in other years after a gain. The continuing data points, however, indicated that, after the crackdown, there were no further gains as there had been in the past. Thus there was evidence for a positive effect of the crackdown.

## Single-Subject/Single-System Design

This design is really a special case of the time-series design. In a single-subject design, responses of an individual are measured over time. Such designs are quite common in treatment research, particularly behavioral interventions, and could be used more often to evaluate other kinds of treatment like physical therapy. More extensive reading on such designs is available in Kratochwill (1978) and Bloom and Fisher (1982). Organizations or systems of any type can be considered subjects or cases in a single-subject design.

In such designs, the baseline period during which there is no treatment or intervention is typically labeled as "A" and treatment periods are labeled "B" and subsequent letters of the alphabet. During each period of baseline and intervention, repeated observations are made. In a *reversal design,* the treatment is temporary, and when it is withdrawn, it is assumed that baseline conditions are reestablished. Observations continue to be made. Such designs are referred to as ABA or ABAB.

Kolko and Rickard-Figueroa (1985) studied the effects of video games on reducing negative side effects of chemotherapy. An ABAB design was used with three male patients. In this study, video games were used as the treatment to provide distraction. For all three patients, video games reduced anticipatory symptoms that returned when games were removed; observed behavioral distress and reported chemotherapy side effects were also reduced. The replication of the baseline and intervention provides a powerful argument that changes are due to the intervention and not to alternative factors.

There are times when it is not feasible to return to baseline. For many treatments, it makes no practical or ethical sense to remove the treatment if it appears to be working. For example, if you were treating a patient who suffered from severe headaches with a stress management protocol and the frequency and severity of those headaches declined dramatically during treatment, you would not withdraw the stress management techniques to determine if the headaches returned. In addition, many treatments are self-sustaining and cannot be withdrawn. It is possible that even if, for research purposes, you wished to withdraw the stress management protocol, the patient would be able to sustain the treatment. Many single-subject designs are, therefore, only AB. If a treatment does not appear to be working or to be having only a slight effect, clinicians are likely to try other treatments and not to return to baseline between each one. Attempting three different treatments would be described as ABCD. With both AB and ABCD designs, it is still possible that the repeated observations under different treatment conditions can be inspected to evaluate effects.

## EXPERIMENTAL DESIGNS

There are two primary characteristics of an experiment: (1) the experimenter controls the treatment or intervention, including when, how, and to whom it is introduced; and (2) study participants are *randomly assigned* to treatment or control groups. The purpose of random assignment is to attain equivalency of groups and to rule out selection as a threat to internal validity. It is assumed that initial differences among participants will be randomly distributed across groups and will not "pile up" in one group. The larger the number of participants, the more statistically valid this assumption is. Although random assignment does not assure initial equivalency of groups, it is the best method for attempting to achieve equivalency. Because the use of control groups and pretests help to control other threats to validity, randomized experiments, which involve all of these controls, present the best evidence that A causes B, that is, they are the most internally valid.

Random assignment is based on the same principles as random selection, which will be discussed in Chapter 5 on sampling. With random assignment, all study participants have an equal chance of being placed in either treatment or control groups. Random assignment cannot involve the judgment of either the experimenter or the subject. It cannot involve choice. It is best done using a method that introduces randomness into the decision, such as flipping a coin to decide whether a participant will be placed in treatment or control group or using a random number table to identify which participants (the first, the fifth, and so on) will be placed in the treatment condition. Methods such as alternating assignments or placing all the morning patients in one condition and all the afternoon patients in the other must be carefully scrutinized for any systematic bias. Morning patients may be different from afternoon patients in some way that could affect the outcome measure.

Although random assignment allows us to assume that persons in different groups will be equivalent, for variables that have a high likelihood of affecting the outcome measure, additional steps can be taken to try to assure equivalency by using *block random assignment*. Within health care settings, patient condition or treatment is often a particularly important variable for such blocking. For example, in our study of chemotherapy emesis treatment, we knew that different chemotherapy protocols cause this reaction to happen more frequently. Because emesis is a major dependent variable, treatment groups differing in this regard would be disastrous. Therefore, a series of random assignments was developed and used for each chemotherapy protocol. This assured equal numbers of patients with each kind of protocol in our treatment and control groups. Similarly, in the BSE study, we knew that BSE instructions are slightly different for women who are postmenopausal or premenopausal. We, therefore, used menopausal status as a blocking variable and randomly assigned to condition within this grouping variable.

The advantages of randomization will be described in two common control group designs. The final section of the chapter will discuss factorial designs that can test whether treatments together have a different effect that is more than a combination of their independent effects, known as an *interaction*.

## Posttest-Only Control Group Design

In this design, study participants are randomly assigned to one of two groups. One group is then exposed to the intervention or treatment and the other is not. Measurement or observation of both groups occurs only after exposure of the experimental or treatment group.

$$R \quad \times \quad 0_1$$
$$R \qquad\quad 0_2$$

This design may be recognized as the "problematic" example of "static group comparison" described earlier with the simple addition of random assignment. The fact that this addition makes the design a respectable experimental design illustrates the power of random assignment. The equivalency between the groups can now be assumed because of randomization. The threat to validity of selection can, therefore, be ruled out. Because time can elapse between randomization and measurement, mortality can become a problem with more participants dropping out of one or the other group before measurement. The longer the time elapsed, the greater this problem can become.

In general, the presence of a control group minimizes the other threats to validity: history, maturation, testing, instrumentation, and regression. It should be noted, however, that although the design appears to be testing the presence or absence of X, in fact, it is testing the presence of X versus whatever else participants in the control condition are experiencing.

## Pretest-Posttest Control Group Design

This design improves upon the previous one by adding another observation prior to the introduction of the treatment. Randomization can also occur after the initial observation although it should not be in any way influenced by it. The importance of randomization is in assignment to the treatment group.

$$R \quad 0_1 \quad \times \quad 0_3$$
$$R \quad 0_2 \qquad\quad 0_4$$

This design may also be recognized as the nonequivalent control group design with randomization added. With randomization, again, equivalency can be assumed. The pretest provides a further check for equivalency. It would be particularly important for small samples. This design attempts to control for all the major threats to internal validity previously described. Mortality, or differential attrition from the groups, should be a continuing concern and will be discussed further in Chapter 5 on sampling.

## Factorial Designs

The experimental designs mentioned so far involve one factor. Typically, we are interested in the effects of more than one variable or intervention. A *fully crossed* factorial design is used to investigate the independent and combined effects of more than one variable. The simplest such design is a 2 × 2 factorial. Example 4.4 illustrates a factorial design in the first BSE study. As can be seen, in a 2 × 2 factorial design testing the presence and absence of each of two factors, four groups are created: one that receives one factor only, one that receives the other factor only, one that receives both, and one that receives neither. The number of cells resulting from a factorial design is calculated by multiplying the levels of each factor so that a 2 × 2 × 2 design would have eight cells while a 4 × 3 × 2 design would have 24 cells. The number of subjects needed, cost, and effort rise dramatically with the addition of each factor or level of factor in such designs. Factorial designs with more than four independent variables are to be avoided as they are cumbersome, costly, and other designs are more manageable for this number of independent variables.

---

*Example 4.4.*
*BSE 2 X 2 Factorial Design*

In the first BSE study, we were interested in the effects of reminders or cues on the frequency of BSE practice (Grady, 1984). We wanted to test two kinds of reminder systems: external cues (operationalized as postcard reminders) and self-managed cues (operationalized as calendars and sticker reminders). Although it would have been possible to test each of these interventions against a control group comparison, it occurred to us that the cues together could have a different effect from a simple combination of their independent effects. For example, if the self-managed cues were extremely successful, the addition of the external cue might have added nothing. On the other hand, the two cues together might have been significantly more powerful than either one alone. We, therefore, adopted a 2 X 2 factorial design as illustrated below:

|  | no postcard | postcard |
| --- | --- | --- |
| no self-management |  |  |
| self-management |  |  |

Whenever studies involve more than one variable, you need to decide whether to investigate them in a fully crossed design. Sometimes such designs produce cells that are impractical, illogical, nonexistent, or unethical. For example, in our studies on patient control, we initially conceptualized "control" as consisting of two factors: information and choice of treatment. When we considered the four cells that would result from crossing these factors, a choice cell with no information presented problems for us. There were potential ethical issues involved in asking patients to make choices without adequate information. Also, we did not believe that such a condition would provide a meaningful sense of control for patients. For our purposes then, we considered the three cells as part of a single factor.

## SUMMARY

Three major types of design are discussed: correlational, quasi-experimental, and experimental. Each is evaluated in terms of internal validity, which allows causation to be inferred. Correlational designs offer the advantage of studying the relationships among many variables, but internal validity is inherently low. Cross-sectional (single-shot), longitudinal, and prospective designs are discussed. The major threats to internal validity are illustrated using two problematic designs: the one-group pretest-posttest design and the static group comparison. Seven threats to validity are described: history, maturation, testing, instrumentation, statistical regression, selection, and mortality. Quasi-experimental designs attempt to control for these threats to validity and are useful when random assignment is not possible. Nonequivalent control groups, multiple control groups with posttest, time-series, and single-subject/single-system designs are described and evaluated. In experimental designs, the experimenter controls the treatment or intervention and randomly assigns participants to condition. Methods of random assignment are discussed. The ability of experimental designs to control for threats to validity is illustrated with posttest-only control group and pretest-posttest control group designs. Basic factorial designs that can investigate more than one independent variable at a time are briefly described.

## EXERCISES

(1) In a survey, researchers found that low cholesterol diets were associated with less heart disease. Make a logical argument that diet causes heart disease. How could longitudinal and prospective designs strengthen the argument?

(2) Health professional students were fainting or getting sick upon their first exposure to severely injured or grossly deformed patients. A videotape was developed to "desensitize" them and lessen such responses. To evaluate this intervention, the students were given an attitude test before and after the videotape's presentation. Evaluation forms were also sent to clinical supervisors to assess how students interacted with these kinds of patients after viewing the videotape.

Discuss the design of this evaluation in terms of the following threats to validity: history, maturation, testing, instrumentation, statistical regression, selection, and mortality. How could the design be improved?

(3) "Heartbreak fatal, researcher claims" is the headline of a newspaper story that says that the stress from severe emotional trauma can lead to heart failure. The findings are based on a study of six heart patients who suffered symptoms such as fainting and irregular heartbeat but showed no evidence of heart defects or disease. All six, however, had experienced severe emotional trauma. This study also shows the episodes respond favorably to certain drugs such as beta blockers.

Critique this study and then design a correlational study to test the hypothesis that heartbreaks are fatal and quasi-experimental and experimental studies to test the hypothesis that beta blockers are effective.

# 5

## *Selecting the Sample*

The purpose of any research project is to discover or test a relationship between two or more variables and also to determine under what conditions the relationship holds. In particular, it is important to be able to *generalize* beyond the specific instances or people studied. Is the finding true for everyone (or most people)? Is it true for all arthritis patients, teenagers, women, people with hand injuries? No one wants to complete a study and only be able to say that the findings hold for the 50 people who came into a particular clinic one Wednesday in 1987. The sample is, of course, only one factor related to generalizability. The nature of your operations, when and where the study is conducted, and other aspects of your procedure are all relevant. The sample selected for study is crucial, however, in terms of the ability to generalize beyond the circumstances of the study, its *external validity*.

Sophisticated sampling techniques can greatly reduce the number of subjects needed for generalization. In fact, political pollsters have raised considerable controversy by their ability to select a few "key precincts," interview a few hundred people, and predict results for elections in which millions have voted, even before all the ballots are cast. Scientific sampling with this degree of accuracy can be conducted by telephone at relatively modest expense once the basic principles are understood. For small research projects and clinical studies, such sampling is not always possible. The basic principles, however, are accessible, and any violations of them can be undertaken with an understanding of the ways in which external validity is consequently reduced.

In this chapter, we shall review several important issues in sampling: how to define the target population and set up screening criteria, issues in defining appropriate control groups, methods of sample selection within the population, choosing the sample size, response rate and attrition, and ethical issues in recruitment.

### DEFINING THE
### POPULATION OF INTEREST

Some questions dictate the sample. A question about reactions to chemotherapy requires a population of patients undergoing chemotherapy. A question about adaptation to chronic illness requires a population of patients who are chronically ill. Whether people use seat belts requires a population of people who have cars equipped with seat belts. Questions about prevention may require a general sample of the population. Whatever the specific requirements of your population, however, you want a population that is representative of the group of interest. It should not be systematically biased in any particular way. For example, patients undergoing chemotherapy include males and females with a range of ages who have a variety of regimens. If your sample included only women ages 30 to 40 on cysplatinum protocols, you would have a highly selected population not representative of cancer chemotherapy patients.

Settings and methods can constrain the population. As discussed in Chapter 2, particular health settings are likely to be populated only by certain kinds of people. Emergency rooms, for example, are more likely to have poor people in them. Each work setting has more of one kind of people than others, men versus women or people of only one level of education and training rather than a range. In general, any particular setting has already *preselected* the population to some extent. It is important to know in what ways the population has been preselected and the ways in which that might affect the hypothesis or your key independent and dependent variables.

### Screening Criteria

Potential subjects do not present themselves to you bearing only the characteristics of interest. They are also of a certain sex, age, socioeconomic status, marital status, and education level. They also may have illnesses or conditions other than the one you are interested in (*comorbidity*). There may be special characteristics that are particularly relevant for your study. For example, whether or not women had menstrual cycles was hypothesized to be related to the difficulty of doing BSE in the BSE compliance studies.

It is important to review sociodemographic characteristics to determine if there are ways in which you want to limit the population. For example, in a study of injuries and work loss, you may only want people with full-time jobs and under age 65. Health status might also be important for that study given that other illnesses or conditions could also cause work loss or even contribute to the likelihood of injuries. You might, therefore, only want people with no other major illnesses. These characteristics would become your screening criteria.

There are also *ethical issues in screening*. People should be able as well as willing to give their consent to research participation. Certain categories are considered ethically at risk: minors (below 18), prisoners, and the mentally disabled or other institutionalized or hospitalized people. When these categories are included in the population being considered, special attention must be given to methods of recruitment to ensure informed consent. These issues will be discussed later in this chapter. The important point here is to determine in advance whether there are ethically at-risk groups in the population.

In deciding characteristics to be used to screen people out of the study, you will be making a number of judgments about the importance to the study of certain subject characteristics. There will be characteristics you judge to be contaminants or distractions to the main question and you may decide to screen on them. There are others you judge important and interesting to the study question, and you may decide to use them to *stratify* the population (discussed below). There are others that may be simply interesting, and you may decide only to collect the information (for example, on age, sex, or number of doctor visits per year) for possible data analysis but not to let it affect your sampling. There are others that you may decide have no relationship to the study (e.g., religion, political party affiliation), and you may ignore them. The elements you ignore contribute to what is called *error variance*. The more such error variance, the harder it will be to find a relationship. The decision about what to ignore is primarily conceptual, and one researcher's question is another's error variance.

Sometimes the decision to ignore characteristics can be a very difficult one that requires a lot of technical or medical knowledge. For example, in treatment studies, small sample sizes may require choosing a *basis for aggregation:* diagnosis or degree of illness or type of medical intervention. It may take a physician or the judgments of several physicians to decide what diagnoses can be grouped together. In a study on recovery from surgery, the type of surgery may have to be ignored or judgments made about similarities between types of surgery. When complex judgments such as these are made, it is useful to record detailed information and to check assumptions after data collection before aggregation is done.

## Defining Appropriate Control Groups

In randomized experimental designs, a sample from a single population is *randomly assigned* to treatment and control groups. There is no need to define separately an appropriate control group. In quasi-experimental designs, however, a control group usually is chosen to test the hypothesis in strongest competition with the study hypothesis. In the study of residents near Three Mile Island (TMI) discussed in Chapter 4, three control groups were chosen (Baum, Gatchel, & Schaeffer, 1983). The study hypothesis was that the partial meltdown at TMI had stressed the nearby residents, which could be demonstrated by scores on psychological, cognitive, and physiological tests. Because it was a posttest-only design, they needed *comparison groups* (an alternative to control groups) for whatever scores they recorded on their tests. If TMI residents recorded very high scores, competing hypotheses might be that most people in the Northeast might have scored that way, that simply living near a nuclear plant might affect scores, or that living near any power plant might have the same effects. They chose control groups to rule out these competing hypotheses.

Control groups are usually matched to the experimental group on variables that are likely to affect the dependent measure. In order to find effects, it is important that control groups be similar to the experimental group in every other way possible that might affect the study outcomes. A corollary assumption is that other variables will not matter, at least not systematically. The particular variables chosen for a "match" and the resulting control groups reflect the theoretical orientation of the researcher. Different fields give different amounts of credibility to competing hypotheses and are likely to ignore different sets of variables. Those with a medical orientation may be more concerned with other physiological or biological factors that could be advanced to explain results; those with a social or behavioral orientation may be more concerned with other social or behavioral explanations. In either case, the unchosen variables may serve as alternative explanations of the findings. Example 5.1 gives a description of just such a controversy.

---

*Example 5.1.*
*What Does a Control Group Control for?*

[Dr. Mary Parlee (1981, p. 639), a psychologist, reports what can happen when an interdisciplinary team gets together to decide on an "appropriate" control group:] A little over a year ago, I was involved in a meeting of biomedical and social scientists concerned with the study of aging. The particular task of this group was to make recommendations concerning the appropriate "control group" of women to be added to a longitudinal study of aging that has been going on for over twenty years with only men as subjects. The male subjects in the aging study are intelligent, highly educated, professionally active and successful, and by a number of psychological and physical criteria they seem to be aging very well. What group of females should be chosen to allow for a comparison of aging in women? The social scientists and biomedical scientists at first met separately to identify the control group. Not surprisingly, the social scientists thought that the sample of women to be added to the study should consist of intelligent, highly educated, professionally active and successful women. If one wants to compare aging in women and men, the reasoning went, of course one would want the two groups to be matched (to be as similar as possible) on those social dimensions that are likely to affect aging. Physiological differences among individuals, from this perspective, are conceptualized as relatively less important. The biomedical scientists, on the other hand, thought that the group of women to be added should consist of the female siblings of the men already in the study. This would maximize the physiological similarity between the two groups and thus, in their view, provide an opportunity to study aging in women and men under relatively "controlled" conditions.

---

## Sampling

Once the target population or *sample frame* has been defined, including any necessary control groups, a sample is drawn from within that population. A detailed discussion of sampling is beyond our scope. Fowler (1984), in this series—Applied Social Research Methods—provides a great deal more coverage of the sampling process. Samples can be drawn in many ways. We shall discuss sampling approaches under three main categories: random samples, samples of convenience, and volunteering.

## Random Samples

A random sample simply means that each person in the population has an equal probability of being sampled. That is, no one member's selection affects the selection of any other. Drawing a sample randomly makes it more likely that the sample will represent the group. It also maintains objectivity and controls any possible researcher bias. As with random assignment to experimental and control conditions (discussed in Chapter 4), random selection is best done using a method that introduces randomness in the process. Even methods that seem unbiased can introduce a bias into selection and undermine the representativeness of the sample. For example, reaching into a file drawer and selecting a few cases may seem random, but in fact, you are not likely to take the first or last file folder.

Selecting a random sample can be a simple one-step procedure, if you have a complete list of the target population, or a multistage procedure starting with some units other than individuals (e.g., housing units or telephone numbers). We shall discuss only sampling from a list. The principles are the same. When a list of the population is available, every person is assigned a number. Then a random number table can be used, taken either from a statistics book or generated by a computer, to identify which members of the population are to be sampled. For example, if you wanted to sample members of a professional group in your state to receive a questionnaire, you might start with the membership directory. If they were not numbered, you would assign numbers. Then, using the random number table, you would pick the identification numbers that matched the random number sequence and send those people your questionnaire.

For a *stratified random sample,* the same procedure is used within each of the subpopulations identified as strata. For your study of members of the professional group, you might decide you want to stratify on degree and sample the Ph.D.s separately from the M.S.s. You would, therefore, assign two sequences of identification numbers and go through the procedure with the random number table twice.

The adequacy of sampling depends on the comprehensiveness of the list. Most lists leave out some people. For example, a membership directory of any professional organization excludes people in the profession who have not joined. Telephone books eliminate people without telephones or with unlisted numbers. These excluded groups can differ in systematic ways from the included groups. Thus it is important to evaluate your list for its completeness.

## Samples of Convenience

These kinds of samples are far more common in research than truly random samples. It is fairly rare to be able to identify the entire population of interest. For example, if you wanted to study people receiving chemotherapy, it would be very unlikely that you could get a list of everyone receiving chemotherapy in the world, the United States, or your own state. You might be able to obtain lists of patients receiving chemotherapy in one hospital or several hospitals. Your hope would be that these patients are representative of chemotherapy patients in other locations. Examining the specific hospital for ways in which the sample

has been preselected for you was discussed in Chapter 2. If it is a
suburban hospital, you may want to sample patients from an urban
hospital or perhaps even include two or three hospitals of each type.

College students, patients in particular practices, women's group
members, people who go to health fairs, assembly line workers in a
particular plant—all these and many more are populations of convenience. They are convenient because they are available to you. You
may not really want to know the health behaviors of college students;
you want to know about health behaviors in general, but you have
access to college students. You certainly do not want to know about the
adaptation to chronic illness of Dr. Jones's and Dr. Arnold's patients
only. In the community BSE study, we were not interested in increasing
the frequency of BSE among women who belong to women's groups,
but women's groups were a convenient place to find groups of women
and to try to recruit them into the study. The assumption is that these
populations of convenience are representative of a larger population or
differ in systematic ways that can be understood and explained. It is a
big assumption, but a generally necessary one in health research.

The method of sampling with a population of convenience is either
going to be random or volunteering. If every member can be identified,
then random selection procedures as described above can be used. If
every member cannot be identified and the number available is very
large, then volunteering, as described below, can be used. If the number
is very small, then you will want to take *every case*. (See Example 5.2.)

---

*Example 5.2.*
*Chasing Every Case*

In the barium X-ray study, we had to devise an elaborate scheme to obtain
a sample of participants. We had access only to one hospital, and the
frequency with which the test was ordered was not high. We, therefore,
literally had to chase every case. Our intervention was providing choice of
preparation options before the test. Because the physician ordered the test
and provided instructions on preparation for it at the same patient visit,
we had to intervene rapidly during that visit, after the physician decided
on the test but before instructions were given. For maximum control, we
wanted our own nurses to provide the instructions.

We outfitted nursing students with beepers like many physicians carry.
They were then paid a small hourly rate to stay nearby, for example, in the
library where they could study. When a physician decided to order the
test, the nursing student was summoned on the beeper and raced to the
patient to recruit him or her into the study and provide the instructions.
The nursing students were also paid a bonus for each patient to encourage
their fleet-footedness between the library and the clinic.

Because the X-ray department keeps records, we were able to tell after the fact if we had missed any cases. We checked each week and assessed where we had gone wrong. If a particular physician had been forgetting to beep us, we had another chat with him or her. After a few weeks of this process, we were enrolling nearly every case. We continued to monitor the X-ray list to assure that no systematic loss of subjects occurred.

## Volunteering

To an extent, volunteering is part of nearly every sample selection. Unless you are using archival data or unobtrusive observation, people who are sampled will still have to volunteer to participate in your study. Volunteering as a primary method of sample selection though is reserved for those cases where there are large numbers of potential participants who are not identified in any systematic way. The only way they come into the study is through volunteering. Methods for recruiting volunteers would include mass media (radio, television, printed notices, recruitment posters, flyers, and so on), direct contact (requests at meetings, telephone calls, and so on), and provider referral.

Volunteers who come forward to participate in your study are motivated by something, and you probably will not know what. If you are evaluating a large program and relying on volunteers to provide data, you are likely to hear only from those who are very positive or very negative about the program. If you are offering a service such as a free laboratory test, you may only recruit people who already know about the test or people who could not afford to receive it in any other way. If you are providing dietetic counseling, the people who volunteer may especially need it and be more responsive than a group selected at random. In general, volunteers may be more likely to be highly motivated because of past experience, to be or to perceive themselves to be at higher risk of the disease in question, or to be people who are generally more health oriented or likely to take personal responsibility for their health. (See Rosenthal & Rosnow, 1969 for a more thorough discussion of ways volunteers differ from nonvolunteers.) Recruitment into the first BSE study relied on patient volunteers with provider referral and showed systematic differences between volunteers and nonvolunteers (Example 5.3).

*Example 5.3.*
*Who Volunteers for a BSE Program?*

In order to provide trained women for possible recruitment into a study, a free BSE teaching program was established in a hospital and offered to patients of two practices (n = 1590) in a letter signed by the physician in charge of each practice and sent about one week prior to a scheduled appointment. Patients were then supposed to be asked at the appointment whether they wanted the teaching. Names of those interested were passed on to the project, and contact was made to set up a teaching appointment. Responses were received for only 64% of the patients, with 8% being ineligible according to our screening criteria, 29% expressing interest, and 27% saying no to the program. Only about half of those expressing interest were ultimately taught and virtually all of those volunteered to be in the study after the teaching.

Because the response rate was so low, it was decided to survey 100 refusers, selected at random, to obtain information about their current BSE, family cancer, health-related attitudes, and demographic characteristics. It was found that study participants differed from refusers in terms of less previous experience with BSE, more family history of cancer, and a longer history of coming to the Health Center. Participants were also less confident that they knew how to do BSE, believed the treatment for breast cancer was more effective, were less fearful or embarrassed about BSE, and were more likely to agree that they were personally responsible for their health (internal health locus of control) and that physicians played an important role in health outcomes (powerful others' health locus of control). Participants and refusers were not statistically different on several demographic items (age, education, number of children) nor on the extent to which they thought about breast cancer, felt personally susceptible to it, or thought fate, luck, or chance controlled health outcomes (chance health locus of control). We concluded that the bases on which these women patients were deciding whether or not to have the teaching were rational. In general, they were self-selecting on need for information, risk, and relevant beliefs. (See Grady et al., 1983, for a complete report of factors affecting volunteering for this project.)

## Sample Size

A commonly asked question is "How many subjects do I need for my study?" For external validity the size of the sample depends on how representative it is. If a random sampling technique has been used and if error variance is low, a relatively small sample can represent the target population. Samples of convenience, whose representativeness is unknown, and samples of volunteers, whose representativeness is unlikely, need to be larger to have any hope of generalizability of findings. As a practical matter, cost as well as other issues of feasibility limit the number of subjects in many studies.

Researchers often worry that they have too few subjects. It is also important to know that you can have too many! With too few subjects, you can fail to find relationships that truly exist in the real world. With too many subjects, you may uncover many more relationships than actually exist in any meaningful way. The importance of sample size can be easily seen by examining tables of statistical significance. As the degrees of freedom (i.e., the sample size) increase, the effect size that is needed to be declared significant decreases. For example, if you only have 10 subjects, you need a Pearson correlation of .58 to be significant at the .05 level, but with 100 subjects, one of .20 is statistically significant. It is important to evaluate statistical significance in terms of clinical or *practical significance*. Is that .20 correlation meaningful given the variables involved? If not, you may wish to adopt a more stringent criterion for statistical significance or specify a level of correlation you consider practically significant.

Using statistical power analyses to determine the sample size needed is often recommended but rarely used. A helpful book on power analyses, geared toward readers with one or two semesters of applied statistics is one by Cohen (1977), which provides power tables for each of the major statistics. Power analyses take into account the *expected effect size*, the *variability of the measure*, and the *significance criterion* to be adopted. With small expected effects and measures that vary considerably (such as blood pressure), larger samples are needed to achieve significance at the traditional .05 level. (See Cooper, 1984, and M. W. Lipsey, 1988, in this series for excellent discussions of effect size.)

There are some *rules of thumb* for the numbers of subjects needed that are related to the statistical tests to be used. For chi-square tests, you must expect at least 5 cases per cell. For multiple regression, there should ideally be 20 times more cases than variables; a suggested minimum is to have at least 4 to 5 times more cases than predictor variables (Tabachnik & Fidell, 1983). For factor analysis, there also should be many more cases than factors. A sample size of 100-200 is good enough for most purposes particularly when subjects are homogeneous and the number of variables is not too large (Tabachnik & Fidell, 1983, p. 379).

## Response Rate/Attrition

The rate at which people respond to being in the study and staying in the study can drastically affect the quality of the sample. Response rate is determined by dividing the number of people agreeing to be in the study by the number of people approached. *Attrition* and *mortality* are terms used to describe dropping out of the study. Even if you have carefully defined the population and adopted a random sampling technique, if response rate is low or attrition is high, the resulting sample will not be representative of the population chosen and results cannot be generalized to that whole population. The more loss from your random sample, the more it will resemble a sample recruited through volunteering.

What is a reasonable response rate? The more carefully selected the sample, the higher the desired response rate. As noted above, a very high response is needed to maintain the integrity of a random sample. Responses from a targeted mailing or a direct request for participation from a sample of convenience should probably be at least 50%. With recruitment through some general advertising source such as a posted notice, response rates cannot be determined because it is impossible to identify the total number of people who saw or received the request to participate.

The important factor in determining the impact of response rate on external validity is not really the percentage of people responding but rather whether there is a systematic bias affecting response. Any information you can gather about possible differences between respondents and nonrespondents should help you evaluate whether there is a systematic bias. Comparisons between the sociodemographics of respondents and the total population might be possible. Close inspection of any clustering of nonrespondents in certain neighborhoods or disease categories or by any other characteristic may uncover bias. Information about response rates and possible bias should be included in reports about the study.

Attrition during the course of the study depends on how long the study is, how self-selected the sample was initially, how much effort is required to continue participation (*respondent burden*), and a host of uncontrollable factors like how mobile the population is. With a highly motivated population and reasonable respondent burden, an attrition rate of only 10% per year is possible. As with response rate, however, the crucial issue in attrition is evaluating the extent to which there is systematic bias. Because the participants have been in the study initially, you should have more data for evaluating whether there is any bias. It is important to examine the reasons for attrition by testing for differences between those who do not complete the study and those who do. To determine the possible impact of attrition, "worst case scenarios" can be tested in which those who did not complete can be treated as though they responded contrary to the desired effect.

## ETHICAL ISSUES IN RECRUITMENT

Ethical issues in research become clearest with recruitment into the study. Naturally, in choosing your research topic and design, you will have thought about any possible negative consequences to research participants. You will have tried to avoid adopting methods that might bring harm to subjects. It is when you face actually explaining the research to a potential participant, however, that the intricacies of the ethical issues become most salient.

The protection of human subjects is not just a personal, moral issue. The United States Department of Health and Human Services has regulations that all recipients of federal grants and contracts must follow. All universities that receive federal grants have Institutional Review Boards (IRBs) to review ethical aspects of research. Most institutions have some review process for grants, not only to protect the participants but also to protect themselves from any liability that might arise from a harmed participant. In addition, many professional organizations have published guidelines (e.g., American Psychological Association, 1982).

The most important and most common form of protection is the participant's signing of an *informed consent* form. Although there are occasions when this form is not necessary or when consent is "implied," it is best to obtain written informed consent under most conditions. It is also wise to have your form and procedures reviewed by the IRB or review committee whether or not it is required. In the excitement of designing and fielding a study, subtle threats to informed consent may go unnoticed by people intimately involved in the project.

### Elements of Informed Consent

There are several types of information that a potential participant should have in order to make an informed decision about whether or not to participate. They should be informed about *the purpose of the study.* This statement can be very general. They should also be informed about *the requirements of the study,* such as how long it will last and what will be expected of them. These statements should be as specific as possible. (Examples of these and other elements of informed consent are presented in Example 5.4.)

The final kind of knowledge that potential participants need is knowledge about *the potential risks* of the research. Risks include physical, psychological, or social injury. Physical injury is self-explanatory, but should be broadly interpreted to include physical stress or potential long-range harmful effects. Psychological injury includes mental stress, which may arise from exposure to events or pictures that instill horror, failure, fear, threats to sexual identity, or emotional shock (Cook, 1976). Social injury includes anything that may hold the participant up to ridicule in the community or in any way threaten her or his standing or reputation.

Consent should be both informed and *voluntary*. It should be clear that the person is free to refuse participation, not only initially but later, and not only to the whole project but to any part of it. Even though withdrawals may ruin your research project, the subject's *right to self-determination* is paramount and must be safeguarded.

A key component to maintaining a participant's privacy and minimizing psychological or social injury is *confidentiality*. Absolute confidentiality is very difficult to guarantee, especially in a longitudinal research project that requires subsequent contacts. There are, however, steps that can be taken to ensure as much privacy as possible. (1) As few people as possible should know the research participants' names. In the BSE project, given that the research assistants made the subsequent contacts, there was no need for the Principle Investigator to ever see participants' names. (2) Identification numbers should be assigned as early in the project as possible. All data should then be discussed in terms of I.D. numbers and not names. (3) In cross-sectional one-shot studies, there is no need to collect names at all. (4) Subjects can generate their own I.D. numbers, making it unnecessary to collect names even in longitudinal studies. A simple set of rules can be used to generate six or eight digit numbers that are easily reproducible by the subject and not recognizable by anyone else, for example, the month of the subject's birth, the middle two digits of his or her social security number, the last two digits of the home telephone number, and/or the year of her or his mother's birth.

---

*Example 5.4.*
*Sample of Informed Consent*

| | |
|---|---|
| Purpose | The Health Care Research Project is interested in ways to help people recover from surgery. |
| Requirements | People who participate in the study will be interviewed twice: approximately one week before and one week after surgery. The interview will take about an hour and |
| Sample | will cover previous experience and beliefs about health |

| | care, physical and mental health, and some general questions about background. After the first interview, they will be given some information about the surgery. |
|---|---|
| Risk | Although you will probably find most of the information helpful, some of it may contain details that are upsetting |
| Right of self-determination | for you. If you object to any part of the information or to any of the interview questions, you may refuse to listen or to answer those questions. You are free to withdraw your consent at any time. Questions will be answered by the research staff at any time during the study. |
| Confidentiality | For the most part, numbers rather than names will be used for program records. A list that contains both the numbers and the names will be kept in a locked file. Any reports about the project will discuss results only in terms of groups without identifying individuals. |
| Reassurance | Your decision to participate or not to participate in this study will in no way affect your health care here at University Hospital. |

* * *

| Consent | I understand the explanation of the Health Care Research Project as given above. I voluntarily consent to participate in this project. |
|---|---|

_____<br>Signature

## Threats to Informed Consent

There are many possible threats to informed consent, either to the information requirement or the voluntary consent provision. We shall focus on the two most common and serious: deception and coercion. For a more complete discussion, see Kimmel's book (1988) in this series.

The major threat to information is *deception*. Deception can take several forms. *Involving people in research without their knowledge or consent* can happen in observational studies or evaluations of an ongoing program. Such studies may not require informed consent if the observation is unobtrusive, anonymity is maintained (subjects names are not known), and the person's experience in the program is not changed in any way. Most times, however, subjects should know that they are in a study, and their informed consent should be obtained.

A common form of deception is *giving misleading information about the true purposes of the study*. If you are conducting an experiment, you may not want subjects to be fully informed about each of the experimental conditions. They should at least be aware that there are different conditions and their general purpose. For example, you probably would not want to say, "We are conducting a stress reduction study. There will be three groups: biofeedback, group therapy, and a control group. You will be randomly assigned to one of these groups." You might say instead, "We are conducting a study on stress reduction. We will be trying different methods with different people." If you are conducting a correlational study, you may not want to be specific about each of your hypotheses. Again, you can generally inform subjects about the purposes of the study. When you judge that you must be somewhat vague to maintain the integrity of the study, it is important to explain the true purposes of the study fully at its conclusion, often called *debriefing*.

Debriefing is even more important when *false information about the purposes of the study* has been given. There are certain kinds of studies that could not be conducted if participants were fully informed about their purposes. In these cases, the researcher invents a "cover story." For example, a study about race relations in a health care team might be described to subjects as a study on group decision making. Such deception should not be undertaken lightly and alternative procedures should be explored. As one noted researcher states:

> The distinction between deceiving others passively by telling only part of the truth versus actively by telling an untruth has little if any moral standing, in our opinion. . . . It brings an additional element into the picture, namely a violation of participants' assumptions that they can trust what the researcher says. (Cook, 1976, p. 213)

If that researcher is also a health care professional, the possible blow to credibility can be even more far-reaching.

The major threat to voluntary consent is *coercion*. Like deception, coercion can be subtle or overt. An investigator may be in a position to *require people to participate,* for example as an employer, a parent, or the head of an institution (a prison, a hospital). Even if the investigator does not have the authority to require consent, the potential participant may perceive such authority. They may feel as though they have little or no ability to refuse. Patients may worry that the health care they have been receiving is contingent on their agreement to participate. Anytime there is some external control of the researcher over the potential participant, there are serious concerns about the person's free will. Special care must be taken to reassure patients that they have the right to refuse.

Another form of coercion is offering incentives or *inducements to participate* that are so strong that the person is unlikely to resist. Money or unaffordable health care can be strong inducements to poor people. Social approval is a strong incentive for most people. Implying in any way that their social standing or esteem depends on cooperation can be an ethically questionable form of inducement. Patients may particularly want to be liked by their health care professionals. Receiving excellent standard treatment in a hospital should not depend on research participation. None of these examples should be taken to mean that no incentives for participation can be offered. Rather, the researcher must be aware of the extent to which certain populations may be especially vulnerable to inducements and take precautions that their freedom of choice is protected.

There is one final threat to informed consent that should at least be mentioned, and that is giving information that people cannot really understand either because it is too technical or it is worded at too high a reading level for the average public. Multisyllabic words, long sentences, and legal jargon (sometimes found in institutional liability clauses) all can make the informed consent form difficult to understand. The final document can be checked for reading level and/or the potential participant can be asked to paraphrase the statements to check for understanding.

## Special Issues in Health Care Settings

In addition to these general concerns about informed consent, there are some special issues that arise in health care settings. We shall briefly discuss three: the capacity of the patient to make choices, the nature of the provider-patient relationship, and the ethics of withholding benefits from control groups.

Patients, particularly ill patients, may have a diminished capacity to make informed choices about research participation. They may be sick or drugged or desperate to find ways to feel better. If their ability to decide is in any way compromised, they should not be asked for consent to participate.

The provider-patient relationship is a privileged one and it is one of unequal power. Providers have no right to give out information about patients, including patient names, without the patient's consent. Therefore, physicians control access to patients and have to lend their support to recruitment. Initial letters about the project usually come from the physician. At the same time, as described above, there can be real or imagined coercion to participate that threatens informed consent. It is important that, at the time of making the decision about participation, the patient understands the separation between the research and the clinical relationship. If the researcher is the provider, it is even more crucial to make this distinction. It is not easy. Confusion about research and clinical roles can lead to other ethical problems. The subject can assume that health problems mentioned to researchers will be passed on to physicians. It is important to remind them that research information is confidential and that they must report health concerns directly to their physicians.

A general ethical issue in research, but one that is particularly acute when studying health care, is withholding benefits from control groups. It is important to distinguish the benefits of standard health care from the hypothesized benefits of an experimental treatment. In no case can the control group receive less than standard health care. They cannot be denied the benefits they would ordinarily receive if they were not in a research study. The hypothesized benefits of an experimental treatment, on the other hand, can be withheld in the interest of determining its effects. If you are convinced (even before the study is conducted) that the experimental treatment is beneficial, it can be provided to the control group after the study has ended.

## SUMMARY

Sophisticated sample selection can greatly reduce the number of subjects needed to make generalizations to a much larger group. The population of interest needs to be defined, screening criteria established, and appropriate control groups specified. Methods of sampling are discussed for random samples, samples of convenience, and samples of volunteers. Sample size depends on the power of the statistical test to be employed, which in turn is affected by the expected effect size, the variability of the measure, and the significance criterion adopted. Response rate and attrition during the study can substantially change the nature of the sample. Ethical issues in recruitment are discussed. The elements of informed consent are reviewed, and threats to informed consent as well as special issues in health care settings are given.

## EXERCISES

(1) For each of the following hypotheses, define the population of interest, screening criteria, and a method for sampling:
  (a) Stress causes flare-ups of rheumatoid arthritis.
  (b) Children who have a parent with them while they are undergoing dental treatment are less likely to be distressed.
  (c) Mandatory seat-belt laws increase the use of seat belts.
(2) Draft informed consent forms as appropriate for each of the samples. Identify any special ethical issues that may be involved and methods of handling them.

# 6

## Choosing Measures and Using Existing Data

Measurement is the heart of scientific research; measurement is what makes it science. Measurement weakness is the most common reason for research failure. Without good measurement, the research results add nothing to our understanding above what could have been achieved with a well-reasoned argument. On the other hand, data that are based on good measurement instruments, collected from a well-defined population, can have a life of their own. They exist whether or not the researcher understands their meaning. That researcher at a later date or another researcher working on another problem at some time may gather up such unexplained research results and tie them together with a previously unthought of explanation. Data stand as the pebbles and rocks in a swamp of speculation.

### CHOOSING MEASURES

Each construct in the design must be measured. If you are comparing healthy to sick people, what is your definition of *healthy*? How will you gather that information? If you want to know whether your health education program appeals more to well-educated people, how will you measure educational level? These kinds of variables are called *independent or predictor variables*. In health research, they usually include sociodemographics (age, sex, race, income, and so on), health history, and other factors directly related to the research question. There are standard and straightforward ways to measure sociodemographic variables, and the more standard the approach, the better because it will make your research comparable to other research being conducted.

Sometimes variables that seem simple to measure will raise unexpected problems. Even very ordinary language can mean different things to different people. For example, in our BSE study, we wished to know whether previous instruction in BSE was related to compliance during the course of the study. We, therefore, asked in the interview, "Have you ever been taught to do BSE before? (If yes) By whom?" Most women said they had been taught at some time; however, they said they had learned from pamphlets or that their physicians had remarked, "Do what I'm doing for yourself about once a month." It surprised us to learn that we had a very different definition of "taught" from many of the respondents. Although they were saying yes, they had been taught, they meant they had been handed a piece of paper or a casual comment had been made suggesting they do BSE. Other respondents, of course, meant what we meant by "taught," a systematic and focused instructional session.

The outcomes of the study, the *dependent or criterion variables,* can also seem easy but become difficult to measure in practice. What is weight loss? Think about this very obvious dependent measure for a moment. What would you use? Pounds lost would be very different for a 350-pound person compared to a 180-pound person. Percentage of body weight is also confounded by overall weight and body type. Muscle weighs more than fat. Some researchers have used displacement, which involves actually immersing the subject in water, in order to determine the fat/muscle ratio. Complicated formulas have been developed by others to represent a more sensitive measure of weight loss than pounds alone. (See Chapter 8 for further discussion of measuring weight.)

Independent variables and dependent variables can be mixed up in health care research. Even within the same study, a single variable will be conceived as an outcome for one set of factors and a predictor for another outcome. Control variables are called control variables merely by virtue of their place in the design.

## Matching Measures to the Research Question

There are some special issues involved in matching measures to research questions, population, and design in health care research. A common problem is deciding just what the outcome is. The study may be designed to change behavior, but the outcome of interest is a change in health status. The simplest example of this is weight loss programs. Weight loss programs focus on some change in behavior such as calorie-counting or using a slow rate of eating or they may focus on some change in cognition or affect such as how one evaluates hunger pains or reacts to depression. The overall goal of this instruction or therapy is the achievement of weight loss. There is really another outcome from the training in, let's say, calorie-counting: the subject engaging in calorie-counting during the program engages in a change in behavior:

Calorie-counting instruction      Calorie-counting        Weight loss

Treatment                      Behavior outcome       Health status
                                                         outcome

The effect of the treatment on the behavior change is not, by itself, very interesting in this example. It would be surprising to learn that instruction in calorie-counting was not related actually to counting calories and would suggest further research on methods of instruction. Similarly, it would be surprising to learn that counting calories and reduction in caloric intake was not related to weight loss. In this example, the most practical and interesting research question is whether those in the instruction group actually lost weight. Engaging in the behavior should also be measured but it functions here as a *manipulation check* that confirms the treatment led to the behavior and that the behavior itself is what is related to weight loss and not some other factor.

A different kind of judgment would be made in a BSE study. Taking the same simplistic design, there would also be two outcomes:

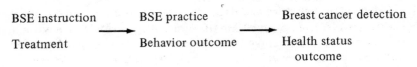

BSE instruction           BSE practice           Breast cancer detection

Treatment                Behavior outcome         Health status
                                                             outcome

The reason BSE is recommended is to improve the early detection of breast cancer. Breast cancer detection, however, presents several problems as an outcome measure. It is so infrequent that the sample would have to be tens of thousands or the study would have to extend for several years in order to have enough cases. A more important problem is that breast cancer is a diagnosis that can be made only on the basis of biopsy results and never on the basis of palpation, whether BSE or clinical breast exam. BSE can only find lumps, thickenings, or changes in the breast. Many of these will not be breast cancer. A few will be. The correct health-status outcome for BSE is the detection of such changes and not the specific diagnosis of breast cancer. Breast cancer detection, though the important health reason for the research, is an inappropriate measure for the research itself. At the same time, there are research questions to be asked about compliance with BSE that focus on the first arrow, the link between treatment and behavior.

## Matching Measures to the Research Population

The research population must be carefully considered when one is choosing measures. One of the most important issues is *respondent burden.* Can these respondents/subjects supply all the information we are requesting? Is there a way to reduce the burden? It is not uncommon to get greedy when you consider all the data you would like to collect. Researchers construct questionnaires that take an hour or more to fill out and interviews that can go on for several hours. In some cases, such requests are reasonable. In others, they are not. An excessive burden is not merely inconsiderate; it also affects the quality of the data. Respondents may become irritated and skip questions or give non-sensical answers. Attitude or affect scales may be biased by subjects' state of irritation or annoyance. Worse yet, they may refuse to respond at all or drop out of the study. Inappropriately heavy burdens may lead to an unacceptably high attrition rate that ruins the entire study.

How does one decide if the burden is reasonable? There are at least two factors to take into account: motivation and ability. The researcher has to make a judgment about how interested the participant is likely to be in the research itself. The activities may be inherently enjoyable or the value of the potential findings high for the participant. If the intrinsic value is not high, compensation may be offered for time or effort. Most research participants, however, provide information solely for the benefit to science or health care. In evaluating motivation, it is important to know how frequently these potential participants are approached for other research projects. People with relatively rare or interesting diseases are likely to be participating in a number of protocols at any given time. Patients in university hospitals may have participated in a number of studies in the past. This experience may affect their willingness to be in your study or their ability to respond because they are already overburdened.

A major ability factor is health. People with arthritis cannot be expected to use a pen or pencil well enough to fill out lengthy questionnaires with open-ended questions. The health of a patient population should always be carefully considered when choosing measurement instruments. In the rheumatoid arthritis study, we wanted patients to complete mailed questionnaires every six months for three years. We precoded all responses so that the patient only had to make a mark on the page in the appropriate box for each question. In addition, we consulted with a secretary in the department who had rheumatoid arthritis as well as the research team members who had clinical experience with these kinds of patients in order to minimize the respondent burden.

Education, particularly reading level, is an ability factor that can influence all your measures, including any instruction. Every piece of written material as well as spoken, such as scripts for interviews, should be evaluated for reading level. There are several simple and standard ways to do this (Dale & Chall, 1948; National Cancer Institute, 1979). The SMOG formula, for example, takes into account the length of the sentences and the density of words with more than two syllables. Other methods also take into account the difficulty of certain words. For a general adult audience, an eighth-grade reading level should not be exceeded.

## Matching Measures to the Design

The issues involved in this match are very similar to those discusses above in terms of the question. The design indicates whether the measures will be tapping independent, dependent, or control variables. In general, the measurement of control variables does not have to be as detailed or sensitive as the others. The most important questions are simply "What do you want to know about? Do you want to measure their health status, their behavior, their psychological or cognitive reactions, or the environment?" These deceptively simple questions are ones only you and your research team can answer. The debate that precedes the decision is an extremely important one, and the research must be undertaken with a clear idea of what the dependent measure is. Drawing a model of the design with an indication of what you want to know is a useful exercise for making you think more concretely.

For example, in the first BSE study, the major dependent measure was health behavior (BSE practice). Another dependent measure was health status (finding any breast changes). Previous research suggested that certain attitudes and beliefs might be related to frequency of BSE practice. The literature also indicated that sociodemographics (e.g., age, education) affected practice and that some of these sociodemographic factors (e.g., age) were also risk factors for breast cancer. We wanted to

TABLE 6.1
Topics for Data Collection in BSE Study

| Time 1 Baseline | Time 2 During Study | Time 3 Follow-Up |
|---|---|---|
| Past health behavior | Health behavior | Health behavior |
| Health status | Health status | Health status |
| Attitudes & beliefs | | Attitudes & beliefs |
| Sociodemographics | | Sociodemographics |
| Environment | | Environment |
| | | Manipulation check |
| | | Threats to validity |

use these sociodemographic factors as predictors in some analyses and as control variables, along with other health-status items and environment, in other analyses. Given that it was a longitudinal, prospective design, we needed to collect the data on the same topics at several points. We sketched out the kinds of data to be collected at baseline, during the study, and at follow-up. At the end of the experimental period, a manipulation check and data about any possible threats to validity were added. We, therefore, had lists of what we wanted to know, as illustrated in Table 6.1.

## Types of Measures

How to collect the data is the next question to be resolved. In the following chapters, we review the major kinds of measurement approaches available. We start in this chapter with existing data because consideration of what might already be available can save time and help you judge what else you might need. We then review self- and other reports, the most common way to collect social and behavioral data. Observational methods and physiological measures are then discussed. Within each of these measurement methods, we give examples of applications of the method to outcomes of the four major types: behavior, cognition and affect, health status, and environment. Once you have decided, for example, that your outcome of interest is cognition and affect, you can skim each of the sections and review the various ways you could collect cognition and affect data. Alternatively, if you have decided on a single questionnaire as your type of measure, you can see what types of data can be collected with it. Table 6.2 gives examples of some of the health-related measures that will be discussed.

TABLE 6.2
Examples of Health-Related Measures

| | *How to Know It* | | | |
| | | | | |
| *What to Know* | *Existing Data* | *Self-Other Reports* | *Observation* | *Physiological Measures* |
|---|---|---|---|---|
| Cognition & affect | hospital admissions for depression requests for pain medication | anxiety depression perceived social support | distress/anxiety | heart rate blood pressure |
| Health behavior | health care utilization work loss | compliance functional ability | pill counts "uptime" | "tracer tags" substance use |
| Health status | patient charts weight no. of heart attacks no. hospital admissions tumor registry | pain visual analogue scale Seriousness of Illness Survey | pain/functional ability mobility | lab tests disease activity |
| Environment | address household composition | life stress social network social climate | home visit observations of health care setting | |

It is important to consider several ways to measure a single construct. As discussed in Chapter 1, "Introduction," every method has inherent weaknesses. By using two or more methods that do not share the same weakness, you can have more confidence in your results. A *triangulation* of methods (see Jick, 1979; Wallston, 1983; Wallston & Grady, 1985) that provides similar or complementary results provides a far stronger case that the finding is a reflection of the "real world." Problems arise, however, when results are not the same. Which results do you believe? Do you believe the increased heart rate, which suggests the subject was anxious, or the self-report of low anxiety? When attempting to assess pain, do you accept the patient's report of extreme pain or the observed low count of pain medications requested? The choice is determined by the quality of the data and, to some extent, your own theoretical orientation.

In each of the sections about methods, we shall review the basic questions about quality of the data. The primary considerations are its *reliability* and *validity*. Reliability means that it is consistent as a measurement tool. Validity concerns whether it measures what it is supposed to measure. A host of factors related to both the inherent properties of the measure and the way it is administered can affect reliability and validity. Our discussion will touch on reliability and validity issues in health care research.

## USING EXISTING DATA

Many types of health data are already collected and stored in hospital or clinic records, patient charts, insurance claim forms, employment records, tumor registries, and other places such as departments of health. It is worthwhile to discover what kinds of records already exist that could aid your research project. Such records may help you to understand the setting, as described in Chapter 2, or the sample, Chapter 5. They may provide an important way to classify your population (an independent variable) or an additional outcome measure (dependent variable). These data have to be reviewed carefully, however, before the decision is made to use them for another purpose.

### Quality of the Data

Evaluating the reliability and validity of existing data depends on a reconstruction of the conditions under which they were collected. Were the data consistently recorded under the same or similar circumstances? Were the data recorded by the same person or someone functioning in the same or similar roles? Are the data a valid measure of what you think they are measuring?

The most important question you can ask in evaluating existing data is "Why were they collected?" If they were collected for a central or necessary purpose of the organization, they are likely to be much more reliable. For example, hospital charges are very reliable. They are virtually always recorded because the hospital must charge for services. They are likely to be recorded by the same person or someone with the same kind of training or background. They also have some built-in checks and balances because they have been reviewed by other people, such as the patient, insurance companies, and/or auditors. Their validity, however, is limited to the reasons they were collected. They are valid indicators of days in the hospital and services performed. Their validity as indicators of health status requires an inferential leap with some understanding that hospital stays are influenced by hospital policy, physician differences, availability of insurance coverage, and posthospital living arrangements. We did find in our surgical study that hospital charges were correlated with nurse ratings of patient illness. The illness data were frequently missing while complete data were available on hospital charges.

Most data collected in health care settings are collected either for financial or for clinical treatment reasons. The financial data, as described above, are likely to be extremely reliable but to have validity of a very narrow sort. Clinical data have both reliability and validity problems; that is, their consistency and meaning are both open to question. They often involve much more judgment and may also be more inconsistently recorded. Their reliability is likely to be influenced by the health professional's clinical judgment, the patient's ability and cooperation, and even the number of patients seen at the facility on the day the data are recorded. Missing data are a very common problem as health professionals in the setting recognize. (See Example 6.1.)

---

*Example 6.1.*
*Patient Charts: "We have it, but . . ."*

A researcher writing a grant proposal needed to include some demographic characteristics of the patients. She approached the physician in charge of the service to request permission either to observe patients in the waiting

room, recording their ages, sex, race, and so on, or to hand out a brief
questionnaire to collect this type of information. "No, no, we have that,"
the physician protested. She rummaged in a file drawer and triumphantly
drew forth a thick interview form. "See? This is the intake interview. We
start out taking all that information. It's right here," she said, pointing to
questions about sex, age, race, income, area of residence as well as length
of time since diagnosis and some health questions. "Isn't this good
enough?" she asked. "It's great!" said the researcher, imagining all the
saved time. Patient charts could be sampled or perhaps even completely
reviewed to summarize all this important information. "So then the
records could be pulled and this information could be coded right off
them," the interviewer mused out loud. "No, no, it's not filled out on most
people's charts," the doctor explained. "We don't have that kind of time."

---

It is fairly easy to see why data based on clinical judgment and chart
notes may be "soft," but laboratory results and X-rays also have
reliability and validity problems. The social or behavioral scientist, who
is outside the system, may too quickly judge these kinds of data as
"hard." Laboratory tests have error rates involving "false positives" and
"false negatives" and require interpretation, sometimes very sophisticated interpretation. The reading of X-rays is a complicated cognitive
skill that requires extensive training and experience. In addition, a
number of factors may affect the quality of the X-ray. For example, the
quality of a mammogram depends on the kind of machine used, careful
maintenance of the machine, the quality of the film, as well as the skill of
the technician, the density of the breast, the cooperation of the patient,
and, finally, the training, experience, and skill of the radiologist making
the interpretation. Clinicians and technicians who have daily experience
with these procedures are aware of such threats to reliability and
validity. Existing clinical data, no matter how "hard" or "soft" they
appear to a social or behavioral scientist outside of the system, should
never be adopted without input from a skilled professional as to their
reliability and validity.

Public health data, like vital statistics, are also subject to biases even
though they have been collected for purposes of research and planning.
Death records, which may seem so absolute, are indeed valid indicators
of death, but the cause of death as recorded may be influenced by many
factors. The attending physician may not know and may guess wrong.
The immediate cause of death (e.g., pneumonia) may be given rather
than the more serious illness that preceded it (e.g., lung cancer). There
are also "rules of thumb" for stating the cause of death. For example,

breast cancer is considered the primary site of cancer and the cause of death if a woman has had it and dies of cancer. It doesn't matter that the breast cancer was four years ago and that bone cancer may have immediately preceded death. Another factor influencing death records is social desirability. Some causes of death such as AIDS or suicide may be embarrassing for family members, and the friendly family doctor may record a more socially desirable reason. Tuberculosis was long considered an illness of the poor and a result of inadequate hygiene. Official records of its frequency as a cause of death as well as its overall incidence during the early twentieth century may seriously underestimate its real rate of occurrence.

Estimates of disease prevalence are virtually always just estimates. Even cancer is not a reportable disease in most states, and statistical estimates are made on the basis of the 14 states that do collect data (Levy, 1985). Abortion rates are completely unavailable prior to 1973 when it was legalized in this country and may still be underreported for certain segments of the population. Suicide involves a complicated judgment with consequences for the family that may be both emotional and financial, affecting the payment of life insurance claims. Careful attention has to be given to the kinds of social, economic, and cultural biases that may influence data that can seem so "official," complete, and accurate.

## Problems of Access

Public health data are, of course, public, and you have the same access to them as any citizen. The library is likely to have national data from the census and the National Center for Health Statistics. Local and state health departments may issue periodic reports and would be the best source for learning what is available. Private health data, however, belong to the organization or institution that collected it, such as hospitals, clinics, insurance companies, and employers. They may have numerous reasons for not wishing to share their data with a researcher. In addition, the relationship between physician and patient is a privileged one, and professional standards may bar your access to patient records. Even knowledge of which patients kept their appointments by name is a sensitive issue because these patients did not waive their privilege and have not agreed to participate in your study. These and related ethical issues are discussed in Chapter 5.

There are several things you can do to make access to records more likely. (1) Be extremely selective in the information you want to know. It is tempting to want to browse through patient records or other clinic files to "get a feel for things." Resist that temptation. Instead, spend extra time beforehand listing the kinds of information that would help your research project and talking to clinic staff about the likely availability, reliability, and validity of such data. (2) Provide the rationale for each kind of information. If you have done your homework, you should have a clear idea of why you need the information and should be able to explain it clearly and in writing if necessary to the people in charge. (3) Create a method of data collection that protects the confidentiality of the patient, such as using identification numbers instead of names. The ethical issues in converting clinical records to research data cannot be stressed too strongly. The data should be separated from identifying information about the patient as rapidly and completely as possible. (4) Use a professional who would ordinarily have access to these types of records to collect the data or to delete identifying information. For example, the receptionist could record the rate at which appointments are broken or the clinical dietitian who conducted the weight loss program could delete names and substitute identification numbers, keeping the only master list that associates them.

## Trying to Turn Existing Data into Research

Instead of having the research question and searching for relevant existing data, there are times when data are available because they were collected for another purpose and someone (perhaps you) wants to turn them into a research project. This approach has been called "have data, will travel" (Martin, 1982). Beware! It is not as easy as it looks. There are likely to be quite serious reliability problems. There may be a lot of missing data. They were probably not collected in the form that would be ideal for data analysis. The wrong questions were probably asked. Reconstructing the conditions under which the data were collected (the methods section of your research project) is extremely difficult. The bottom line is that post hoc research lacks the controls of real research. It is better to consider existing data a beginning for a research project, not an end in itself.

There are some things you can do to improve the situation. First, try to find out everything that was done when the data were being collected, including who collected it, how, where, and why. Second, determine how the "subjects" were recruited. Third, develop a question. Don't just fish around analyzing data, hoping that an interesting finding will emerge and that you will notice it. Fourth, collect more data. For example, if you have clinical data from a weight loss program, design a follow-up. None of these steps will make existing data an ideal research project, but they may help develop a very good pilot study or a decent clinical evaluation.

## EXISTING DATA ON
## COGNITION AND AFFECT

This area has the least amount of existing data, and it is likely to be quite poor. There may be notes in the patient's chart indicating the clinician's judgment that the patient was depressed or irritable. There may be a record of hospital admissions for depression or some other affective disorder. Many things, however, may influence whether a clinician makes such a note or a hospital admission is ordered. In addition, there may be some information that could be interpreted as related to cognition or affect. For example, Langer, Janis, and Wolfer (1975) used requests for painkillers as a measure of psychological reactions to surgery. The behavior of asking for pain medication could be indicative of many things aside from actual pain, however, like stoicism or beliefs about the medication.

## EXISTING DATA ON BEHAVIOR

There are several types of patient behavior that are reflected in existing records in hospitals, clinics, or practices of various kinds: utilization of services, appointment-keeping, medication compliance, and other forms of treatment compliance. Insurance company records can indicate seat-belt use from accident reports. Employer records include work loss or sick leave information. Health clubs have utilization records. Pharmacies keep track of the reordering of medication. Uncovering these data and determining how they might fit into your research project is a creative process. We shall give a couple of examples.

## Utilization

Use of services can be analyzed from either the organization's or the patient's viewpoint. The facility may want to know which services are used and how frequently in order to facilitate planning for the future. A utilization review can be vital in completing a *needs assessment*. It is surprising how frequently social and behavioral researchers overlook this useful form of information. (See Example 6.2.)

---

*Example 6.2.*
*Needs Assessment:*
*Figuring Out What They Really Want*

At a large university health service, a new health educator was hired to initiate some health education programs that would respond to the needs of the students as well as faculty and staff. Naturally, she began with a "needs assessment." She designed questionnaires to be distributed to each of the groups asking them which services they used and which new ones they would like. When her first group, the faculty, returned only 8% of the questionnaires, she engaged the help of a graphic designer to prepare a more attractive questionnaire booklet for her next groups. Unfortunately, the response rate from the students was even worse. She was extremely discouraged. How could she meet the needs of these people if they wouldn't tell her what their needs were?

At the same time, the women's clinic of student health services was booked for the rest of the semester with students who wanted birth control information, and sex education seminars were always crowded and sometimes had to turn people away. An assessment of service utilization patterns should have been the first step in the needs assessment. Students were telling her their needs by "voting with their feet" rather than filling out questionnaires. Probably because of her training in a single narrow method for doing needs assessment, she focused on paper-and-pencil measures rather than this easy and obvious behavioral measure of demand.

---

## Appointment-Keeping

Keeping appointments is a basic measure of compliance with treatment regimens. With many kinds of diseases and conditions, regular appointments are recommended. These appointments may be with the physician or nurse practitioner, or they may be for blood work or other laboratory tests, or they may be auxiliary appointments with dietitians, physical therapists, or other allied health professionals. Compliance with keeping these appointments may be an important indicator of the extent to which the patient is following doctor's orders. In addition, the facility itself may be interested in appointment-keeping as part of an overall evaluation of their success in health care delivery. Every service has a usual "break-rate," which is the number of appointments that are canceled, rescheduled, or simply not kept. Some services may want to keep track of their break-rate while they experiment with different forms of call backs or change other aspects of their procedures.

An issue related to appointment-keeping is *program attendance* for programs that are scheduled to go on for a period of time, such as weight loss programs or exercise classes or smoking cessation clinics. The attrition rate for such programs can be extremely high. For health professionals who want to evaluate the effectiveness of their particular technique of health behavior change, this drop-out phenomenon is a real nuisance. Sometimes these people are simply dropped from the data analysis, and the program is evaluated only for those people who actually completed it. Sometimes the outcome measure is adjusted for length of time in the program. Program attendance itself, however, can be an important way to evaluate the acceptability of the program. It doesn't matter how good the program is if people will not come and take advantage of it.

## EXISTING DATA ON
## HEALTH OUTCOME/STATUS

This area has the most amount of existing data in health settings. Patient records have as their primary purpose the recording of health-status data and are an obvious source. They include things like weight, the occurrence of heart attacks, and health history. Laboratory results recorded there can indicate disease activity in chronic diseases like rheumatoid arthritis or lupus. Less obvious are other kinds of clinic or hospital records such as length of stay in the hospital and number of admissions. Then there are incidence of disease records for reportable diseases like venereal disease or cancer. Finally, there are vital statistics like death records.

## EXISTING DATA ON ENVIRONMENT

Many of the kinds of existing data on specific health care settings have been reviewed in Chapter 2, "Health Care Settings and Collaborative Research." These settings are the environment in which you may want to collect data or in which data may have already been collected. In addition, you can find out some very rudimentary things about the potential subject's environment from information in patient records. Addresses can tell you whether they live in urban, suburban, or rural areas. Census information can tell you more about these areas. Patient records may also provide information about household composition— the social environment of the person.

## SUMMARY

Measurement is the heart of scientific research. Choosing measures involves several steps. Measures must be matched to the research question, the research population, and the research design. What you want to know is discussed in terms of four major topics: cognition and affect, health behavior, health status, and environment. How to collect data in each of these areas is discussed in terms of four types of measures: existing data, self-reports, observation, and physiological measures. A table is provided to summarize examples of the kinds of data that can be collected using these measures for these topics.

Existing data, such as health or hospital records, can be used to classify the population or the setting or an independent/predictor or dependent/criterion variables. The quality of the data needs to be carefully evaluated. Problems of access to records can be made easier by being selective and specific, protecting confidentiality, and using health professionals for data collection. The pitfalls of trying to turn existing data into research are discussed. Examples are provided of existing data on cognition and affect, behavior, health status, and environment.

## EXERCISES

(1) In the study on "heartbreak" described in exercise 3 of Chapter 4, sketch out what kinds of information you would like to collect on cognition and affect, health behavior, health status, and environment. (Refer to Table 6.2.) Identify the independent and dependent (predictor and criterion) variables.

(2) If you were to devise a study about factors affecting recovery from surgery, what data from hospital records would be useful to collect?

# 7

## *Self-Report and Other Report*

### GENERAL ISSUES

You want to know whether patients are taking their medicine, whether they liked the treatment program, whether they were anxious before surgery or depressed afterward, whether their condition has improved after treatment, or whether they have friends and relatives to help them during recovery. In other words, you want to know something about their behavior, cognition and affect, health status, or environment. How do you find out? The answer is deceptively simple—ask them. Their answers are called "self-reports."

If research were in fact that simple, there would be no need for methods books like this. What you ask, how you ask, whom you ask, and who asks can crucially affect the quality of your data. Fortunately, there are other researchers, many with special training in psychometrics, who have spent considerable time developing scales that will measure many of the constructs you wish to research. Later in this chapter, we shall review some of the existing measures that are frequently used in health research.

Self- and other reports are often referred to as "paper-and-pencil" measures, but they can also be administered in an interview format, either face-to-face or by telephone. While individual subjects are usually asked to report about themselves, there are times when others are needed to provide reports about subjects' behavior, mood, or health functioning. Patients may at times be unable to provide data, or reports from others (sometimes termed *informants*) may supplement data provided by patients. Family members are useful informants about patient functioning at home, while nurses' ratings of patient discomfort may be a more realistic way to collect systematic data than asking a postoperative patient to keep a log. Information supplied by informants is called "other reports."

Health status is frequently assessed by asking nurses or physicians to make a judgment about a patient's health. To make these judgments, they may utilize physiological data, observations of the patient, and/or patient self-reports. Overall, however, health professionals are giving you their best clinical judgment when making such a rating. If you are not a clinician yourself, familiar with the health issues involved, you may need to know more about how such clinical judgments are formed and what data are considered. You should find out if there are standard categories, scales, or units of judgment for the disease of interest. For example, in designing a lupus study, we had to become familiar with the clinical and laboratory manifestations of the disease that physicians use to judge disease activity and severity. These kind of data had to be collected along with the physician judgment of how the patient was doing. It is also important to note that the same care must be taken in designing a report form for other reports as for self-reports. The issues discussed in this chapter should be considered relevant for all such reports.

## Biases

A major problem in self-reports, and to some extent in informant reports, is whether the respondent is telling the truth. Bias can enter into self-reports consciously or unconsciously. *Social desirability* is a major contaminant. Respondents often know, or think they know, what a "good" answer would be. They know that "good patients" take their medicine, aren't afraid or depressed, and get better. They may subtly (or blatantly) bias their responses in this "good" direction because they want to be "good patients." Respondents may also know, or think they know, the hypothesis of the study. They may then bias their responses to be "good subjects" and confirm the hypothesis or, if they disagree with it, they may bias their responses in the other direction. It is important to note that these biases can be very subtle. Subjects are not lying when they merely portray a somewhat flattering picture of themselves. Respondents may also be inaccurate because they *forget* what happened. Means of enhancing accurate recall will be discussed in the section on behavior.

Another subtle bias in self-reports is *social comparison*. Many questions call upon the respondent to make judgments. For example, as a patient, in a follow-up interview sometime after surgery, one of us was asked, "Overall, on a 10-point scale, how are you doing?" Being a researcher, I asked, "Compared to what?" I would say different things if I were comparing myself to my ideal of health, to the sickest I was prior to the surgery, to other patients I might have known following surgery, or to how I felt right after the surgery. Patients do make social comparisons (Taylor, Wood, & Lichtman, 1983), and we need to be aware of the influence this may have on responses to our questions.

## Scale Development

Although many people do it, it is inappropriate merely to write some items and assume they measure the construct of interest. For any self-report instrument, *reliability* and *validity* should be documented. This can be a lengthy and cumbersome process. See Example 7.1 for a description of the years of work on a single instrument.

Reliability answers the question: Is the measurement consistent? This takes two forms. Is it internally consistent? Do the series of items "hang together" and measure a single construct? Internal consistency is usually assessed and reported in terms of Cronbach's *alpha reliability* with values from 0 to 1. In general, .60 is viewed as minimum acceptable alpha for a scale. It is also important that responses to an instrument are consistent over time, called *test-retest reliability.*

When an instrument is determined to be reliable, we then must consider whether it measures what it purports to measure—is it valid? Whether it appears to be upon reading is *face validity,* but this is typically not sufficient. How it relates to other measures of the same construct reflects *construct validity.* Whether it is sufficiently different from measures of other constructs is the question of *discriminant validity.* If the results found with the instrument are consistent with theory, it is said to have *predictive validity.*

The details of instrument development and validation are beyond the scope of our specific coverage. See Nunnally (1978) for further discussions of scale validation. As a minimum, it is important to pay attention to item writing, to start with many more items that are needed, to obtain initial data on appropriate populations, to write items that tap the construct, and to collect validation data. Some examples of scale validation relevant to health care may provide insight into the process (Bergner, Bobbitt, Carter, & Gilson, 1981; Smith et al., 1984; Zonderman, Heft, & Costa, 1985).

*Example 7.1.*
*Developing Health*
*Locus of Control Scales*

In 1972, we were asked to evaluate a diabetes education program being conducted by an interdisciplinary team. After discussing program goals with the health professionals, we observed the series of classes. As we went through the program, it became clear to us that a central focus was getting people to take responsibility for what happened to their diabetes. This concept seemed parallel to the construct of internal locus of control typically assessed with the I-E Scale (Lefcourt, 1966; Rotter, 1966). That scale distinguished internal locus of control or personal responsibility from external locus of control or responsibility that was attributed to fate, luck, chance, or powerful others. People who scored "more internal" had been found to be more active in attempting to control their outcomes. Such an orientation seemed to be the goal of the diabetes education program.

Because Social Learning Theory (Rotter, Chance, & Phares, 1972)—the theory upon which the construct of locus of control was developed—postulated that measurement of expectancies should be as specific as possible, we decided to develop a scale to measure locus of control over health. We wrote 34 items as face valid measures of generalized expectancies of control with respect to health. We administered those items to nearly 100 college students and used their data to select items (1) on which there was variability, (2) that formed an internally reliable scale, and (3) that balanced the direction of wording. The resulting 11-item Health Locus of Control (HLC) scale showed initial construct and discriminant validity through a low positive (.33) correlation with the original I-E Scale. Thus there was sufficient overlap to argue that our new scale measured locus of control, but sufficient difference to suggest that the scale was in some way unique (Wallston, Wallston, Kaplan, & Maides, 1976).

We conducted two further studies to show predictive validity. We were able to show that subjects who valued health highly and who held internal health locus of control beliefs sought more health information than other groups as was predicted by theory. Furthermore, these results were not found with the general I-E Scale, suggesting further discriminant validity. We also showed that participants in weight reduction programs that were consistent with their locus of control beliefs were more satisfied than mismatched groups. We also showed that scores on the HLC Scale were stable over time. It was four years of work before the new scale and supporting data were published.

In the meantime, other work had been done suggesting that locus of control was really a multidimensional construct (Collins, 1974). The work of Levenson (1981) distinguishing between chance and powerful others externality seemed particularly relevant to health care. We found that our 11-item scale had 5 internal items, 5 chance external items, and only 1 powerful others item. We, therefore, again went through the scale development process. We developed items reflecting the three dimensions to form an item pool of 81 items. We tested the items using persons waiting at the airport. Using similar criteria, we developed two forms of the Multidimensional Health Locus of Control (MHLC) Scales, each with three 6-item subscales representing the dimensions of chance externality, powerful others externality, and internality. Again, we showed sufficient internal consistency and relationship with existing scales. Correlations with health status were used to show initial predictive validity. We published these new scales in 1978, but we noted, "The extent of the validity and reliability of these instruments will not be fully known until they are appropriately used in a number of studies (Wallston, Wallston, & DeVellis, 1978, p. 169). The development and refinement of such scales is a lengthy and, to some extent, never-ending process.

---

## Finding Out What Exists

Before you even consider scale development, you should find out what scales and measures exist in the literature. Sudman and Bradburn (1985) give detailed instructions for tracking down existing survey questions. There are also some general sources worth checking. Ward and Lindeman (1978) provide a compilation of nursing research instruments. They provide descriptions and critiques of 140 psychosocial instruments, most of which are included in the volumes. Other measure compilations are cited in specific sections of this chapter. More of the existing measures and reviews of measures are of affect and cognition than of behavior or health status, although a growing number of self-report indicators of health status and behavior are being developed (Kaplan, 1985).

If you can't find reviews of existing instruments appropriate to your variable, another good source of measures is journal articles. Flip through recent issues in the most appropriate journals or initiate a computer search to see how other people have measured the same construct. But beware; just because other people have used a technique does not mean it is good. You need to evaluate it. But starting with someone else's measure is typically faster and almost always easier than starting from scratch.

## Instrument Selection

If you have found an instrument that has published data indicating it is sufficiently reliable and valid, there are other issues you must consider before you select it. Is it simple to administer? Will its length fit with your procedures? Is it clear? How intrusive is it? Will respondents likely be angered or exhausted by completing the instrument (Green, 1985)?

What about the level of language? Many instruments have been developed for use primarily with college students. They may reflect language that is not comprehensible to your subjects. (See Chapter 6 on matching measures to the research population.) Scales also may have items that are age-inappropriate or irrelevant to your population. For example, in a study of persons with epilepsy, we omitted an item related to driving from a locus of control scale given that persons with this condition are typically instructed not to drive.

Even if you think the content is appropriate, you must consider whether your subjects will view it as appropriate. For example, in a study of persons with rheumatoid arthritis (RA), we included a general locus of control scale. A number of people left out these items. In our next questionnaire administration (this is a longitudinal study), we wrote an extended letter answering common questions, including "Why do you want to know about the 'psychological stuff'? What does that have to do with RA?" This approach was far more successful in generating responses than just including the scale that wasn't face valid to our respondents.

After all of these criteria have been considered, you should have an idea of the most appropriate measure for your use. This will often involve trade-offs. For example, you may have to go with a longer instrument to obtain a valid one.

## Adapting Existing Instruments

If no instrument you have located is perfect for your use, you may be able to change an instrument so that it better fits your needs. This is still preferable to starting from scratch. Remember that, if you are changing an instrument, you must reestablish reliability and validity. Copyrighted scales generally cannot be changed, but you can discuss it with the owner.

The most common adaptation is shortening a scale. You can often get assistance with this by calling the scale developer and asking for the best items. You should select items that correlate well with the total scale, that represent the range of scale content and wording, where possible. In the BSE study, for example, we used 4-item versions of the 6-item MHLC subscales.

When you can obtain the data on which the original scale was developed, the shortened scale can be checked for reliability and validity by reanalyzing the original data. For example, the Desire for Control Scale we developed (Smith, Wallston, Wallston, Forsberg, & King, 1984) was 14 items. We were using many instruments in our field experiments, so a shortened version was desirable. We did new analyses showing that a 7-item version was internally consistent and discriminated among the known groups used for the original validation (B.S. Wallston et al., in press). Many researchers will make their data available to you if you contact them.

Another common adaptation is a change in response options. Likert scales, for example, ask to what extent the respondent agrees or disagrees with a statement. Minor changes in the number of response options available rarely affect the validity or reliability of the scale. Using five, six, or seven responses from strongly agree to strongly disagree is fairly arbitrary and such change may facilitate integration with the rest of your questionnaire. Changing to a strictly yes/no or true/false format, however, while easier for respondents, will greatly decrease the scale range and is likely to affect other scale properties.

Tampering with question wording is far more problematic than other kinds of changes. New validity and reliability data *must* be collected. You may, however, want to do this to fit your needs. A general questionnaire might be more useful if it were specific to your population. For example, Holroyd et al. (1984) used the 36 items from the two forms of the MHLC, but in each item, *headache* was substituted for *health* in their study of cognitive effects of biofeedback training for headache sufferers. Be very careful about minor wording changes in items. They can affect how respondents interpret an item and thus scale validity. Using a very different sample from the ones the scale developers used can also require new validation.

## SELF- AND OTHER REPORTS OF
## COGNITION AND AFFECT

Only by asking people can we tell how they feel (affect) or what they think (cognition). While there are techniques to detect cognitive processes with measures such as reaction time, the *content* of cognition cannot be observed directly. Self-report measures thus provide the most direct assessment possible of both affect and cognition.

There are many existing scales for measuring cognition (including attitudes and beliefs) and affect (including mental health status). Robinson and Shaver (1973) provide a review of measures of self-concept, values, attitudes toward people, sociopolitical attitudes, and religious attitudes. They include the actual measures, assessments of reliability and validity, and sources for further information. Kaplan (1985) reviews techniques for measuring quality of life. Green (1985) reviews a number of self-report instruments in terms of their effectiveness for use in medical settings. There are also numerous sources of instruments not directly related to health research that may prove helpful, especially for mental health assessment (e.g., Chun, Cobb, & French, 1975; Comrey, Backer, & Glaser, 1973). A few instruments that are frequently used are highlighted here.

*State-Trait Anxiety Inventory (STAI).* The STAI is among the most common instruments used to assess affect. Developed to assess anxiety, one series of questions asks for feelings *right now*, or *state anxiety*, while the other asks how the individual generally feels, or *trait anxiety* (Spielberger, Gorsuch, & Lushene, 1970). Validation and normative data utilized college and clinical samples.

*Center for Epidemiological Studies Depression Scale (CES-D).* This is a 20-item scale that measures depression (Radloff, 1977). It was developed for use with a general as opposed to a clinical sample, but it does include vegetative state items (e.g., I did not feel like eating) as well as mood items (e.g., I felt sad). Respondents are asked the frequency of these feelings/behaviors over the past week on a one to four scale.

*Multidimensional Health Locus of Control Scale (MHLC).* Locus of control is a belief or cognition about the connection or contingency between behavior and outcomes. The MHLC Scales (Wallston et al., 1978) consist of three 6-item subscales measuring beliefs in control by chance, powerful others, or the self (internal). Responses are on 6-point Likert-type (i.e., strongly disagree to strongly agree) scales. Reviews of studies provide clear evidence of scale reliability and some validity evidence (Wallston & Wallston, 1981, 1982). It is important to consider whether locus of control is theoretically relevant before using it in research. There is more validity evidence for use of the locus of control construct in research on persons with chronic illness (Roskam, 1985, provides a review) than for use in prevention research (Wallston & Wallston, 1981).

*Krantz Health Opinion Survey (HOS).* There are two subscales measuring preference for self-treatment and involvement with 9 items, and preference for information about health care with 7 items (Krantz, Baum, & Wideman, 1980). A true-false response format is used. There is good evidence of internal consistency and test-retest reliability. Validity has been shown with college students (Krantz et al., 1980). The information subscale using a Likert format has also been validated across three adult samples (Smith et al., 1984).

## SELF- AND
## OTHER REPORTS OF BEHAVIOR

Because behavior is difficult and costly to observe, it is often necessary to settle for self-report information on behavior. There are some techniques that can be used to improve the validity of such self-reports, but caution must always be used in interpreting such data. Because behavior is often the dependent variable of interest, careful attention should be given to its measurement.

Under "General Issues," we discussed aspects of self-report bias. Bias can enter into self-report consciously, in terms of attempts to look good, and nonconsciously, in terms of forgetting or other misrepresentation. Specificity of questions and short time spans can help decrease invalidity due to forgetting. It is easier to answer the question, "What did you eat yesterday?" than to respond accurately to questions about "usual" diet habits. Asking participants to keep a log of behavior may be a particularly helpful approach to improving accuracy. Even if completed only once a day, such records are superior to recall of the past week.

Self-monitoring (in the form of a log or diary) produces a representative sample of behavior not accessible to observers and avoids the problems of retrospective reporting. It may be *reactive*, however. That is, the act of monitoring a behavior can alter its frequency. To improve the accuracy of self-monitoring: (1) it must be easy to do, (2) target behaviors should be as concrete as possible, (3) forms should be portable and small enough to fit in a pocket, (4) respondents need to be carefully instructed, (5) the forms should require brief and not excessively intrusive responses, and (6) some system of reminders or salient cues for easy timing should be developed (e.g., associating recording with meal times) (Turk & Kerns, 1985).

Attempts to look good may be more difficult to avoid. Framing questions to make it clear that behavior is acceptable, however, may help. When asking about failure to comply with medication regimen, we asked, "Some people sometimes do not take their medication when they are supposed to. How often did you skip taking your arthritis medication during the past month?" We tried to make it clear that skipping medication was a common occurrence to decrease the sense that it was "bad" and shouldn't be reported. (See Example 7.2 for another approach.)

---

*Example 7.2.*
*Obtaining Self-Reports of BSE*

In the BSE studies, we wanted a measure of BSE practice that went beyond the usual self-reported frequency in response to the question, "How many BSEs have you done in the past six months?" Particularly because we were planning to reward subjects for each BSE, the pressure to overreport would be great. The first strategy adopted was to make it a little more difficult to report socially desirable behavior. Subjects were asked to fill out a response form monthly to indicate whether or not they had done a BSE. If the response was yes, then several other questions needed to be answered, for example, "How long did it take?," "Where did you do it?," and so on. The premise was that it is more difficult to tell several lies than one.

A serendipitous event caused us to change strategies. One of the researchers herself was asked by a nurse practitioner if she did BSE. When she hesitatingly said yes, sort of, the nurse then asked which of her breasts was larger (like hands and feet, a common occurrence). If she had been performing high-quality BSEs, she would have been able to answer this question easily (she couldn't). It then occurred to us that we could focus on information that subjects would know only if they had engaged in the action. We created the BSE Record, which has a schematic drawing of the breast for noting findings during the self-examination. It is printed on carbonless "snap-aparts" so that an automatic copy can be made and sent in as evidence that a BSE was done. In other words, the Record creates a "behavioral residue" that can be measured. The trouble of filling out the record and making up answers to a series of questions should deter most people from faking "good" responses and improve the accuracy of the self-report behavior.

---

Even though self-reports of behavior have problems, they are likely to be more valid than asking for *behavioral intentions* (e.g., "How many lectures on arthritis have you attended in the past six months?" versus "Would you go to a lecture on arthritis if it were available?"). A direct lie on recent past behavior is not extremely likely, while it is easy to convince yourself you would behave in a socially desirable way given the opportunity. There are also data to suggest the validity of self-reports of behavior (Haskell, Taylor, Wood, Schrott, & Heiss, 1980).

There are not very many existing indices for self-reports of behavior although some behavioral items are often included in general instruments. For example, questions about behavior as a response to pain are usually included in assessments of pain; in this chapter, we have classified pain as primarily a health-status issue. Questions about social activity are often included in measures of social support, which we shall discuss in terms of the environment. Other behavioral items are developed for specific studies and are generally not available as an instrument.

Some instruments of functional ability, conceptualized as indicators of health status or quality of life, actually call for self-reports of behavior. To the extent that you are interested in actual health status, a second level of inference is involved. Not only are there issues of the accuracy of self-reports as discussed above, but also the issues of the extent to which the behaviors reflect health or illness. Some people keep going irrespective of symptoms. Others easily take on the "sick role," stopping much typical activity. Such characteristic response to symptoms or illness clearly limits the ability to infer health from behavior. We shall describe two such measures of functional ability before turning to a discussion of the measurement of the quite well-known behavior pattern, Type A behavior.

*Sickness Impact Profile (SIP).* This is probably the most widely used measure of behavior in the face of illness (Kaplan, 1985). It is a lengthy instrument (132 items) with subscales reflecting sleep and rest, eating, work, home management, recreation and pastimes, ambulation, mobility, body care and movement, social interaction, alertness behavior, and communication behavior (Bergner et al., 1981). Respondents agree or disagree with each item. Scale values, based on judges' ratings of dysfunction, are used to weight items. The SIP has shown impressive reliability and validity, correlating with self-assessments and clinical ratings (Kaplan, 1985).

*Arthritis Impact Measurement Scale (AIMS)*. This scale is intended to measure functional status of patients with rheumatoid arthritis (Meenan, Gertman, & Mason, 1982). Scales for mobility, physical activity, and activities of daily living are included in the 67-item inventory. The AIMS correlates with physician ratings of health status and discriminant validity of subscales has been shown (Kaplan, 1985).

*Type A Behavior Pattern (TABP)*. While originally assessed with a structured interview that included ratings of behavior during the interview (Friedman & Rosenman, 1974), there are now several self-report inventories to tap coronary-prone behavior. The Jenkins Activity Survey (JAS) (Jenkins, Zyzanski, & Rosenman, 1979) is the most commonly used measure. The 52-item self-report inventory typically takes 15-20 minutes to administer. While there is clear evidence of validity for this instrument, the JAS does not predict coronary heart disease as well as the structured interview (Turk & Kerns, 1985).

## SELF- AND OTHER REPORTS OF
## HEALTH STATUS

Self-report is an indirect method for assessing health status. There do exist, however, systematic surveys that are used to assess morbidity. Reeder, Ramacher, and Gorelnick (1976) include scales and indices of health status, health behavior, utilization of health services, and health orientations. They provide descriptions and copies of the instruments. Ware, Brook, Davies, and Lohr (1981) provide information for selecting health-status measures.

A common indicator of health status is pain, a variable researchers often want to measure. Pain, however, is conceptually complicated. It is fundamentally a private cognitive and affective experience. Given the same "objective" level of pain, individuals may experience it quite differently and express quite different levels on rating scales. The amount of pain an individual is experiencing can also be inferred from pain behaviors, such as the amount of time standing or walking (*uptime,* Sanders, 1980) or the amount of medication ingested. These behavioral aspects of pain can also be assessed through self-report, but again individuals may vary for reasons other than the amount of pain experienced. Self-reports can only provide indirect assessments of pain intensity. The pain experience overall includes cognitive, affective, sensory, behavioral, and physiochemical elements, and multimodal assessment of the entire pain context is essential (Karoly, 1985). In this section, we shall describe two common instruments for measuring pain as well as two overall measures of health status.

*Visual Analog Pain Scale.* This scale is quite commonly used to assess pain intensity. An unmarked 10-centimeter line is anchored at the ends from "no pain" to "pain as bad as it could be" and respondents give their subjective perception of pain along the line (Bradley et al., 1981; Huskisson, 1974).

*McGill Pain Questionnaire (MPQ).* This questionnaire provides multidimensional assessment of the quality of pain using verbal description (Melzack, 1975). It has been widely used and appears reliable and valid (Bradley et al., 1981). Keefe (1982), however, discusses problems in terms of response constraints.

*Seriousness of Illness Survey.* This survey (Wyler, Masuda, & Holmes, 1968) is a self-report checklist of 126 symptoms and diseases. A severity weight is provided for each item based on degree of discomfort, disability, life threat, duration, and prognosis to create a single health-status score.

*Karnofsky Performance Status.* This is a scale that has been used in cancer research for observer report of health status (see Grieco & Long, 1984). Physicians (or others) are asked to assign a percentage score from 0 to 100 where 0 is dead and 100 is normal with no evidence of disease. There is a description for each 10-point interval. The subjective judgments required may be unreliable (Kaplan, 1985). Scale scores, however, are correlated with survival in lung cancer (e.g., Stanley, 1980). Recent work by Grieco and Long (1984) shows improved reliability when observers are trained on the KPS using more system-atized procedures. It is, however, important to note that physicians may systematically underestimate the impact of illness on quality of life by missing much of the daily dysfunction (Kaplan, 1985).

## SELF- AND
## OTHER REPORTS OF ENVIRONMENT

The environment includes not only the physical environment but the social environment. Both can be important in affecting health status and outcomes. The physical environment can sometimes be directly assessed through observation, but often this method is too costly or not possible. Self-reports of treatment settings have been developed and are described below. The social environment almost always depends on self-report. Measures of the social environment can range from simple questions about household composition (the number of people living in the household, their ages, and relationships to the study participant) to elaborate measures of social support.

Social support is conceptualized in two important ways: the amount or structure of support and the quality or functions of support. When social support is conceptualized in terms of its structure (instead of its functions), it is typically referred to as a social network and is considered a part of the individual's environment. The presence or absence of relationships, the number of people in the network, and the interrelationships of the people (termed *density*) are typical network measures (Moos, 1985). When social support is conceptualized as a person's perception of the quality/availability of support or the quantity/adequacy of support, it is in the cognitive/affective domain. It still represents an assessment of the social environment, however. There are numerous measures of the perceived availability of support, none of which is sufficiently validated as to be preferred over the others (House & Kahn, 1985). In this section, we shall describe one frequently used measure of social network and one of social support.

Another aspect of the environment that has received considerable attention in health research is stressful life events. It has been noted clinically for decades that illness follows on the heels of a major life stressor, such as divorce or the death of a loved one (see Dohrenwend, Krasnoff, Askenasy, & Dohrenwend, 1982, for a history of this research). Stress caused by such events is generally considered a challenge to the individual's ability to adapt, both physically and psychologically. The assessment of environmental events that serve as stressors has been a major research focus and has created much measurement controversy (e.g., Dohrenwend & Dohrenwend, 1978; Sandler & Guenther, 1985). We shall briefly describe the Dohrenwends' scale, although interested researchers should also examine the Holmes and Rahe (1967) Social Readjustment Rating Scale.

*Ward Atmosphere Scale/Community-Oriented Programs Environment Scale.* Moos (1985) has developed instruments that can be used to describe the characteristics of hospital-based and community-based (Community-Oriented Programs Environment Scale) treatment settings. They assess the quality of interpersonal relationships, the program goals, and the nature of the program structure. Examples of use include studies of hemodialysis units (Rhodes, 1981) and oncology units (Alexy, 1981-1982) in hospitals.

*Social Network Index.* Berkman and Syme's (1979) 4-item Social Network Index combines self-reports of behavior and affect. Items include marital status, the number of friends and relatives "you feel close to," the frequency of contacts with friends and relatives, and church membership and other group associations. Responses to these items are then combined in a complicated formula to provide a single score of an individual's social network.

*Interpersonal Support Evaluation List (ISEL).* This is a 40-item scale developed by Cohen (Cohen, Marmelstein, Kamarck, & Hoberman, 1985). The ISEL has subscales for four kinds of support: tangible, appraisal, self-esteem, and belonging. The latter three kinds are highly correlated and seem to represent forms of emotional support. The tangible/emotional distinction and even broader distinctions among support functions may be particularly important in health research, because different types of support may affect health outcomes in different ways (Wallston, Alagna, DeVellis, & DeVellis, 1983; Wortman & Conway, 1985).

*Psychiatric Epidemiology Research Interview (PERI).* This instrument contains 102 life events that reflect different domains (e.g., work, family, finances) and both positive and negative events (Dohrenwend & Dohrenwend, 1978; Dohrenwend, Krasnoff, Askenasy, & Dohrenwend, 1978, 1982). Respondents indicate whether each of the events has occurred in their lives during some defined time period. Developed as an interview, the instrument can also be used in questionnaires. When used as a measure of stress, weightings of the stressfulness of various events are often used. Most comparisons show, however, that weighting does not significantly improve prediction over the sum of negative events (Kale & Stenmark, 1983).

## SUMMARY

Self- and other reports include paper-and-pencil measures like questionnaires as well as interviews. Almost any kind of data can be collected by simply asking subjects. Major biases include social desirability, forgetting, and social comparison. Scale development is a lengthy and cumbersome process, better undertaken by people with special training and skills. There are, however, many existing scales that have been published along with reliability and validity data. Tips are given for finding, choosing, and adapting these scales. Examples are provided of scales to measure cognition and affect, health behavior, health status, and environment.

## EXERCISES

(1) Read a couple of the original articles and compare the reliability and validity of two scales that measure the same or similar constructs (e.g., anxiety/depression, functional disability, social support). What are the limitations of each of the measures? Under what conditions would you use each of the scales?

(2) Devise a self-report form for reporting daily food consumption. Include quantity as well as features of the environment (where, when, with whom). Test it on yourself for at least two days.

# 8

## Observation and Physiological Measures

### OBSERVATION

Rather than rely on self-reports of behavior, which can be biased and distorted, why not observe behavior directly? It is more complicated than it sounds. In fact, creating instruments for the collection of observational data can present all the same problems as creating scales for self-reports. Observers share some of the same biases as subjects, who can be viewed as observers of themselves. There are, therefore, reliability and validity problems as well as reactivity, a problem caused by the presence of an observer. These issues will be discussed in this chapter.

An additional issue is that there are many things that do not lend themselves to observation. Cognition and affect cannot be observed directly. Many health-related behaviors are low frequency, for example, taking a pill four times a day. Other behaviors are generally done in private, like breast self-examination. It would be expensive and obtrusive to try to observe these kinds of behavior. There are, however, *unobtrusive measures* that provide indirect evidence that the behavior occurred. These will also be discussed as a form of observation.

### Observational Categories and Systems

Categories determine the behavior that will be observed out of an ongoing stream of behavior. The system determines how that behavior will be sampled. Are you interested in its simple occurrence/non-occurrence? Are you interested in its duration? Is it a low frequency behavior or a high frequency behavior? Do you want to know what immediately precedes or follows it? Answers to these questions will determine whether you want to sample events or time frames.

How you construct categories and set up a system of data collection determines the quality of the observational method. Category selection is a form of theory construction (Viet, 1978). It is a way of structuring the possible alternatives. Some researchers suggest informal observation at the outset before categories are tightly constrained. It is also important to test your method to see whether the observational system works. With the availability of more sophisticated equipment, complex observational schemes are becoming more feasible because data can be fed directly into a computer. It is important to remember, however, that simple observations may also provide useful measures.

Several people have suggested criteria for the development of categories and systems (e.g., Bickman, 1976; Gellert, 1955; Weick, 1968). There are some general considerations that should be taken into account in any system. Categories should be

(1) *derived from the problem/theory* being investigated; the system should be relevant to the question under study;
(2) *narrow*, designed to focus on selected aspects of behavior;
(3) *objective*, with a small amount of inference required for classifying behavior and little information needed about the surrounding context to categorize the behavior;
(4) *clear*, explicitly defined, specific enough to distinguish important differences in behavior but general enough to keep the number of discriminations to a minimum;
(5) *complete*, exhaustive of the type of behavior recorded;
(6) *distinct*, with as little overlap as possible; and
(7) *easy*, recorded rapidly and simply, preferably with check marks or strokes rather than words.

## Reactivity

The act of observing is likely to affect the behavior of those being observed, that is, it is likely to be reactive. Persons might behave in a more socially desirable manner when they are being observed. Chronic pain patients might show less (or more) pain behavior than when they are alone. Dental patients might demonstrate a more careful and thorough technique of toothbrushing or flossing when observed by the hygienist. People drive their cars more slowly on holiday weekends when they know they are more likely to be observed by police. All of these are examples of reactivity to observation.

Several factors are related to the degree of reactivity associated with observation. Smith, McPhail, and Pickens (1975) showed that proximity to observers was important in increasing the reactivity of those observed. Time helps habituate people to observers. It isn't clear whether the actual presence of observers causes more or less reactivity than electronic equipment, like radio transmitters and videotape recorders. Spender, Corcoran, Allen, Chinsky, and Viet (1974), however, found more socially desirable responses when videotape was used than when one or two observers were present in the setting.

Clearly, obtrusiveness is an important problem in observation and there are not easy solutions because of the ethics of concealment. The use of unobtrusive measures deals specifically with the issue of reactivity (Webb et al., 1966). Unobtrusive measures focus on the consequences of behavior, that is, changes in the environment that occur if the behavior takes place. For example, there will be fewer pills in the pill bottle if the patient has been taking the medication. With most unobtrusive measures, however, there are major validity problems. There are often good alternative explanations for the environmental change. For example, the patient may have thrown the medication away or someone else may have taken it.

## Reliability

With observational measures, reliability is seen as the agreement between two observers viewing and recording the same events. *Interobserver agreement,* then, is a more precise defining term. Indices of such interobserver agreement can be calculated in a variety of ways. One possibility is simple percentage agreement, the number of agreements divided by the sum of the agreements and disagreements. Alternatively, rather than considering individual items, the total frequencies of agreement could be compared. This is a far less stringent procedure. The first method is the most commonly used.

A major problem that is often ignored is that percentage agreement can be quite misleading when some behaviors occur frequently and others infrequently. For example, 2 out of 3 correct on category X leads to 67% agreement and 19 out of 20 on category Y leads to 95% agreement. In each case, there is only one tally different. In addition to this issue, percentage agreement provides no correction for chance agreement between observers.

There are several indices that do correct for chance agreement. Cohen's Kappa (Cohen, 1960) estimates the degree to which chance agreement has been exceeded when comparing two observational records. The proportion of agreement to be expected by chance is based on the observed marginal distribution for each category for each pair of observers, somewhat analogous to chi-square. Light has extended Cohen's Kappa to permit easier comparisons between multiple observers (Light, 1971). These indices are preferable to simple percentage agreement, particularly when one of the behaviors is much more frequent than the others.

Reliability assessment itself is quite reactive, that is, observers may behave differently in the presence of an observer of *their* behavior! It is critical to assess reliability over the course of the study and, where possible, for observers not to be aware when reliability is being assessed. There have been several studies of observer reliability issues by Reid and his colleagues. In one study, Reid (1970) found that when observers were told that their observations would be checked against a standard, they demonstrated greater agreement with the standard than when they were led to believe their observations would not be checked. In another study, Taplin and Reid (1973) compared three schedules of reliability monitoring. They actually did continuous monitoring but told observers different things. They found the highest average reliability when observers were told they were being monitored covertly on randomly chosen occasions; there was lower average reliability when observers were aware they were being monitored on specific occasions. The lowest average reliability resulted when observers were told they would not be monitored. These results suggest that random, covert monitoring is most effective in encouraging reliability.

Obviously, the training of the observers and the nature of the coding scheme, particularly its complexity, will also affect reliability. It is also important to have the coding scheme clearly recorded in writing. This will facilitate the task of the observers and provide a convenient reference when the research is being analyzed and written for publication.

## Validity

The validity of observational data is an issue that is rarely raised. It is difficult to assess. The best approach appears to be multiple measurement procedures. It is difficult to find known external criteria for observational data. Just because such data are reliable, that is not sufficient to assume they are valid. Is the observation measuring what you think it is measuring? The *level of inference* involved in the observation is one factor that can influence data validity. For example, rating a behavior like crying would seem to be a valid measure of crying;

however, rating a general affective state like fear might not be a valid measure of fear. The observer is inferring that a pattern of behaviors are indicating the person is experiencing fear; the person might actually label his or her own emotional state quite differently.

## OBSERVATIONAL MEASURES OF COGNITION AND AFFECT

### Distress/Anxiety

Observational measures of distress and anxiety always involve inference about internal emotional states based on external manifestations. In most cases, these measures focus on coding behavior (as discussed below in the section "Pain Behavior"). In some cases, they also include judgments about internal states. There are some scales that attempt to provide semiobjective ratings of behaviors assumed to be related to stress and anxiety. As examples of such measures, Zung and Cavenar (1981) discuss the Hamilton Anxiety Scale (Hamilton, 1959) and the Anxiety Status Inventory (Zung, 1971).

Venham, Bengston, and Cipes (1977) used an observational measure in conjunction with heart rate and a child's self-report measure of distress to assess children's responses to dental visits. Three independent judges viewed videotapes of the visits and gave each child a rating from 0 to 6 on a clinical anxiety scale and a cooperative behavior scale for each of three periods that corresponded to specific dental procedures. The anxiety scale involves considerable judgment about the child's level of distress. For example, category 3 is described as follows: "Shows reluctance to enter situation, difficulty in correctly assessing situational threat. Pronounced verbal protest, crying. Protest out of proportion to threat. Copes with situation with great reluctance." Despite the amount of judgment required of the observer, interobserver reliabilities ranging from .78 to .98 are reported. The anxiety ratings also showed the same pattern of findings as the heart rate measure.

### OBSERVATIONAL MEASURES OF BEHAVIOR

### Pain Behavior

As noted in Chapter 7, the pain experience is multifaceted. Pain as a subjective experience has been distinguished from pain behavior

(Fordyce, 1976). We have discussed pain primarily in terms of health status. It is pain behavior that can be observed and coded, however, and there have been several successful attempts to do so with patients with chronic low back pain. Keefe and Block (1982) used five nonverbal pain behaviors (sighing, grimacing, rubbing, bracing, and guarding) in an observational system that was tested using videotapes of subjects walking, sitting, standing, and reclining. The system showed adequate interobserver reliability and its validity was tested by correlations with pain ratings of both patients and naive observers, responsiveness to operant treatment, and successful discrimination between pain patients and normal and depressed subjects.

Kulich, Follick, and Conger (1983) developed a much longer list of pain behaviors. They also videotaped chronic pain patients, but rather than imposing categories they had developed, the researchers had the patients, their significant others, and four experienced physicians view the videotapes and nominate the behaviors they thought characterized pain. They came up with a total of 2105 behaviors, which they organized into 80 categories. Two independent raters then classified the behaviors into the categories to test the coding scheme.

Follick, Ahearn, and Aberger (1985) then further refined this pain behavior taxonomy and examined its reliability and discriminant validity. They used a 16-category system for trained raters to view videotapes, recording pain behaviors at 20-second intervals. Setting a standard of greater than 69% interobserver agreement, they selected seven categories for discriminant analysis between the group of pain patients and hospital worker controls. Four categories (partial movement, limitation statements, sounds, and position shifts) accounted for 75% of the variance in group membership and correctly classified 94% of the pain patients and 95% of the controls. On a second sample, these same four categories correctly classified 89% of the subjects. One of the limitations of this line of research is that it is only with chronic low back pain patients; a different set of categories may discriminate people with other kinds of chronic pain.

## Compliance

There are few aspects of compliance with health behavior that can be observed directly. Seat-belt use has been observed (Robertson, 1975; Robertson, O'Neill, & Wixom, 1972; Robertson et al., 1974). In one clever study of the effects of media messages on seat-belt use (Robertson et al., 1974), residents of certain neighborhoods receiving various messages by cable television were observed and a follow-up interview was conducted. Observers stood at carefully chosen sites and recorded with a small hand-held tape recorder the driver's sex, racial appearance (because race itself cannot be directly observed), and approximate age as the automobile approached. They then noted whether or not lap or shoulder belts were being used as the car passed and also recorded the license plate number for tracing to obtain the interview (Kelley, 1979). The results of this complex study were clear-cut: There were no effects for the media campaign. The care with which the observational method was implemented made the authors quite confident in their conclusions.

More common in compliance research are indirect measures that are used to infer that the behavior has occurred. In medication compliance, pill counts and prescription renewals have been used (see Cluss & Epstein, 1985; and Gordis, 1979, for reviews). In order to control for the possibility of falsification, some researchers have done unannounced pill counts or tried to assure that patients were unaware of the count (Boyd et al., 1974; Haynes et al., 1976; Linkewich et al., 1974; Sharpe & Mikeal, 1974). Others have used pill counts as only one measure in combination with physiological measures or interviews. In general, interview data overestimate compliance measured by pill count. For example, Park and Lipman (1964) found that, of 100 patients who classified themselves as compliant with imipramine therapy, pill count classified only 57 as compliant. On the other hand, pill counts overestimated compliance measured by a physiological test. For example, Bergman and Werner (1963) found that by day nine of a penicillin regimen, 18% of the children could be classified as compliant by pill count but only 8% by a urine test.

## OBSERVATIONAL MEASURES OF HEALTH STATUS

### Pain/Functional Ability

Karoly (1985) suggests several *unobtrusive measures* of pain "products and consequences" based on Webb et al. (1981). These may also more generally be seen as measures of *functional ability*. For example, the amount of pain a patient is experiencing may be inferred from the wear on his or her cane or shoes or home exercise equipment. The inference is that a person experiencing pain will be less mobile and less wear will be evident. The kinds of books and articles in a patient's personal library or the collection of medications in a pain patient's medicine cabinet may suggest an effort to cope with pain and, therefore, how much pain is being experienced. Any or all of these "products and consequences" provide indirect evidence of pain and how the patient is functioning.

In a study on operant treatment of back pain, several measures of functional ability were taken (Cairns & Pasino, 1977). The amount of time in-patients spent walking or riding an exercycle was recorded. In addition, an unobtrusive measure of "uptime" was used. A microswitch was placed under the mattress of the bed and connected to an event recorder that inconspicuously collected data about the number of times patients got in and out of bed and the number of hours spent out of bed. It is clear that these measures would be highly correlated because one must get out of bed to walk or ride the exercycle. Nonetheless, the use of three measures strengthened the researchers' conclusion that functional ability responded to operant conditioning (positive verbal reinforcement). All three measures showed the same pattern of results.

There are many clinical measures of functional ability that can be used in research. For example, in physical therapy, there are measures of mobility and flexibility—*range of motion* measures—that can be used in arthritis research. There is also mechanical equipment, ranging from the simple exercycle to the cybex, which can measure exercise duration, effort, and physiological effects simultaneously. The distinction between observational and physiological measures of health status is fairly arbitrary given that clinical judgments of health status often depend on observation.

### Seizures and Other Infrequent Events

In a study on behavior modification of seizures, observers were used to identify both seizures and preseizure behavior in children (Zlutnick, Mayville, & Moffat, 1975). Two trained observers or one observer and a parent watched the child for one hour or more from opposite sides of the room noting the time and occurrence of each seizure. The study design called for a baseline record of the frequency of seizures, followed by an intervention (shaking the child) in the preseizure phase, and a postintervention observation of the frequency of seizures.

Two observers were used in order to increase the likelihood that each seizure was counted. Because the two observers might not agree, it was important to calculate a measure of interobserver agreement. With a low frequency event like seizures, however, the calculation of agreement presents some problems. At first, the researchers in this study used the standard measure of agreement (agreements/agreements + disagreements). They soon noted that perfect reliability could be obtained in the absence of seizures and that the importance of disagreement about the occurrence of a seizure was minimized with this formula. Because agreement on the identification of seizures was central to the study, reliability checks were not computed until at least six seizures had been noted.

## PHYSIOLOGICAL MEASURES

### General Issues

While we often consider physiological indices to be "hard" data, issues of reliability and validity must be considered just as with other kinds of measurement. In general, social scientists are not well trained in the use of physiological measurement. If you are a social or behavioral scientist, you should involve a collaborator or consultant unless you have special expertise. Clinicians in the health field are trained in the use of physiological measures. A major role played on our research team by nurse and physician collaborators is in sharing their expertise around these measurement issues.

It is important for clinicians to be aware that standards for research and clinical use of a measure may be somewhat different. Often for clinical use, measures are used in a categorical way. You are concerned that someone's lab values are in a range that determines a disease and you want that determination of the disease to be reliable, but you do not care a great deal about the exact value. As a researcher, you want a sensitive dependent measure that you can use *parametrically*—that is, the value itself is important and you want that to be reliable. Often, therefore, in research, you will want to take multiple measures of the same indicator, such as blood pressure, and use the average of those values as your variable, because averaging across instances produces more reliable measurement. Because there is a great deal of individual variability in physiological indicators, where possible and appropriate, you can take baseline measurements and look for changes from baseline that are related to your independent variable.

A general issue relevant to determining validity of the physiological measure you select is the *specificity* of that measure in relation to your dependent variable of interest. Is the measure measuring what you think it is measuring? For example, is heart rate a valid measure of anxiety or could it be indicating another kind of arousal? This issue is discussed further in the next section on cognition and affect.

Irrespective of validity, physiological measures can be useful in conjunction with self-report as a means of increasing the validity of self-report measures. A now classic social psychological study used a fake physiological measure as a "bogus pipeline" to emotional reactions. Subjects were wired to a complex electronic device that they were told could measure true positive or negative feelings. Under this condition, subjects' self-reports of unpopular beliefs were increased (Jones & Sigall, 1971). This finding suggests that the knowledge that physiological indicators of behavior will be assessed may increase the accuracy of self-reports of such behavior. For example, using a saliva test to measure smoking behavior in conjunction with self-reports may increase the likelihood that subjects will give a more accurate report of their smoking behavior.

## PHYSIOLOGICAL MEASURES OF
## COGNITION AND AFFECT

### Stress/Distress

The most common use of physiological data in health psychology is to assess the level of *stress or distress*. Distress is the cognitive and affective response to stress, that is, the individual's psychological response. Physiological measures that assess either organ or system functions in the body (e.g., respiration, muscle tension) and biochemical measures that assess endocrine system activity (e.g., catecholamine and corticosteroid secretion; Baum, Grunberg, & Singer, 1982) are measures of arousal. The nature of the arousal (anger, anxiety, sexual excitement) cannot typically be determined from the physiological indicators. To assume that muscle tension, for example, is a measure of anxiety is clearly inferential, because "psychophysiological responses are not linked invariantly to psychological or behavioral states" (Cacioppo, Petty, & Marshall-Goodell, 1985, p. 289).

Another classic study in social psychology by Schacter and Singer (1962) demonstrated that arousal may be mislabeled in response to contextual cues. Epinephrine, a drug that increases arousal (including heart rate) was given to subjects, only some of whom were told the typical effects of the drug. All subjects then interacted with a humorous confederate. Subjects who were not told the effects of the drug and those given false information about its effects reported more euphoria than those who could explain their arousal as a side effect of the drug. A parallel study induced reports of anger in subjects. Thus it has been argued that emotional experience depends on both physiological arousal and an appropriate label for that arousal. To the extent that this is the case, expecting to detect the affect by measuring only the arousal omits an important part of the process of emotional experience.

Catecholamine assays are used by some researchers to measure stress. While it is argued by some that "increased levels of catecholamine in urine or blood samples serve as reliable indicators of stress" (Palinkas, 1985, p. 68), if *distress* is of interest, such measures are clearly inferential. The details of using catecholamine assays are beyond our scope here. Baum et al. (1982) provide a more thorough discussion. A few of the reliability issues are worth noting, however, because they provide examples of the kinds of issues to be considered in all physiological measurement. Factors such as activity level and ingestion of coffee, alcohol, or tobacco affect catecholamine levels, and their influence must be considered in data interpretation. Time of day and circadian rhythms affect excretion, so time must be controlled in data collection. Because of tremendous individual variability, baseline measures are recommended where possible. Preservatives and refrigeration are critical for urine assay. Plasma has rapid fluctuation and catecholamines in the blood have a half-life of less than one minute, so getting an accurate measure from blood is quite difficult.

In justifying inferences from physiological indicators, the logic of the argument that a particular affect and not others is present is important to consider. Multiple operations (i.e., different indices) of the common conceptual variable help make the case for construct validity. For example, let us consider an experiment where the experimental group receives information about the sensations they can expect during a surgical procedure and the control group receives no such information. If heart rate, blood pressure, and respiration all show reductions in the experimental group while high arousal continues in the control group, the inference that there is reduced distress for the experimental group is stronger than if only a single measure had been used.

## PHYSIOLOGICAL MEASURES OF BEHAVIOR

Physiological indicators are often used to assess various aspects of compliance. It is important to remember that when behavior such as dieting is of interest, weight loss is only an indirect indicator that dieting has occurred. Only by inference can conclusions be drawn about eating or exercise behavior.

### Smoking

Biochemical indicators of smoking behavior include thiocyanate (SCN), expired air carbon monoxide (CO), blood carboxyhemoglobin (COHb), blood or urine measures of nicotine, and cotinine (from blood, urine, or saliva). Bliss and O'Connell (1984) provide an excellent review of the issues involved in using these measures. Their review forms the basis for this discussion.

Thiocyanate (SCN) is the most commonly used biochemical index because of its low cost, reportedly long half-life, and ease of sampling. SCN can be assayed from plasma, serum, or saliva. Typically, a cutoff point is established to determine smoking abstinence. Numerous studies have shown little overlap between the level of SCN among smokers and nonsmokers. False negatives (smokers with a negative test) range from 5% to 19%, and false positives (nonsmokers with a positive test) from 2% to 19%. Bliss and O'Connell describe several drawbacks to this measure. SCN is not very good for detecting light smoking. Although it had been seen as a major advantage of SCN that it is eliminated slowly from the body, careful review of the literature suggests that the half-life may range from one day to over two weeks. Therefore, temporarily abstinent smokers may also be false negatives. A major disadvantage of SCN is that other factors affect SCN levels, thereby contributing to false positives. Differences in flow of saliva, diet (including almonds, cabbage, broccoli, and cauliflower), workplace exposure to cyanide, and gender all may affect SCN rate and create false positives.

Other measures of smoking have even more serious problems, according to Bliss and O'Connell. Nicotine, COHb, and CO all have half-lives under four hours so abstinence will invalidate these measures for detecting smokers. Cotinine appears to be quite sensitive (low false negatives) and specific (low false positives) but it is usually more expensive than SCN. Nicotine levels in the cigarette may affect cotinine.

Bliss and O'Connell (1984) suggest that biochemical indicators should always be used in conjunction with self-report, and where these disagree, a secondary biochemical indicator could be added. They recommend SCN with cotinine as the secondary indicator.

## Weight Control

Body composition provides an indirect assessment of behavioral efforts such as diet and exercise. Stewart, Brook, and Kane (1980) provide a review of measures of the condition of being overweight. All measures of weight or fatness appear to be related to health.

Measures of skin-fold thickness appear to be valid indicators of body fat. Skin-fold is measured at three points, and equations exist (Siri, 1956) to calculate percentage of body fat. Interrater reliability needs to be established and test-retest reliability by a single rater should also be checked (Dickson-Parnell & Zeichner, 1985).

If weight is measured, the reliability of the scale is essential. Relative weight may be used rather than actual weight. Relative weight is the percentage of weight in relation to average weight given age, sex, and height. The Metropolitan Life Tables frequently used to determine average weight are of questionable reliability (Stewart et al., 1980). The National Health Examination Survey is a better source (see U.S. Bureau of the Census, 1985).

An alternative to relative weight that is slightly preferable is to calculate weight (W) in some relation to height (H). This is called a power index (Stewart et al., 1980). For men, the most valid power index appears to be $W/H^2$. For women, $W/H$ or $W/H^{1.5}$ appears better. These indices do not take into account large bone structure or muscles, so some people may inappropriately appear overweight. One means of comparing power indices is to assess the extent to which they are independent of height.

## Substance Use

Both to assess medication compliance and substance abuse, physiological indicators may prove helpful. Obviously, the specific substance will determine the nature of the indicator, and it is impossible to review those here because there are so many. Examples are given to illustrate the methodological issues.

Serum assays on blood samples may provide accurate assessments of whether subjects have ingested medication (or other substances) (Cluss & Epstein, 1985). Drugs vary in the rate of absorption and metabolism, however, so timing of blood drawing is very important. Body weight and other factors may also influence measurement. Such assays are also time-consuming, expensive, and are an invasive procedure that may not be agreeable to subjects if done only for research purposes.

Urine assays also provide a direct indicator of recent drug ingestion. Again, knowledge of the absorption and excretion patterns are critical for accurate assessment (Cluss & Epstein, 1985).

For compliance, tracer "tags" may be added to medication and tested through urine assay (Cluss & Epstein, 1985) because simple, inexpensive drug assays are not available for many common drug regimens. Riboflavin meets the requirements of an ideal tracer substance, because it is inexpensive and nontoxic. It is present in many foods and in nonprescription vitamins, however, so outside ingestion can invalidate its use as a compliance indicator if these other sources are not assessed. A series of studies was conducted to evaluate the accuracy of urine ultraviolet fluorescent tests for riboflavin (Dubbert et al., 1985). These tests can be reliable and valid if doses of 50 milligrams of riboflavin are used, and observers are trained to use a matching to sample observation procedure. They can only assess medication taken within eight hours, however.

## PHYSIOLOGICAL MEASURES OF HEALTH STATUS/OUTCOME

Physiological indicators are an important source of information on health status. It is likely to be the dependent variable of interest to health professionals. In considering whether health status is relevant or appropriate as your dependent measure, however, you need to consider whether your independent variable or treatment is sufficiently powerful to affect health status. If you expect to have an indirect effect on health status mediated by behavior or affect, you should measure the mediators as well as the final health outcome to test the entire chain.

It is also important to select the physiological measures most appropriate to the health/disease issue of interest. If you do not have technical expertise, you should seek it out to make this determination. *Disease a Month* is a helpful journal that provides comprehensive information on a different disease each month.

*Mortality.* Death is certainly a powerful dependent variable. However, under most circumstances, the incidence is so low that a very large sample will be necessary to have sufficient power to detect differences between groups in mortality. Although, as already discussed, there are many problems with validity of *cause* of death obtained from death certificates, the fact of death is highly reliable and valid under most circumstances.

Because death is likely to be low incidence, you may instead want to focus on years of survival. For many diseases, data exist on probability of survival or case fatality rate. These can provide a basis for comparison with your samples, in addition to your between-group comparisons.

*Morbidity.* Comprehensive physical exams including complete biochemistry and EEG workup provide the most valid indicators of disease status (Palinkas, 1985). Nonetheless, there are serious problems in reliable diagnosis and classification of illness, as most health professionals are well aware (Kaplan, 1985).

*Blood pressure.* Because of its relative ease of measurement, blood pressure is probably the most frequently used physiological indicator in health psychology research. It is typical practice to improve reliability by taking three readings and using the average recording (Palinkas, 1985). Of course, blood pressure is the critical measure when hypertension is of interest. Validity is an issue, however, because cutoff levels vary across studies from 140/190 mmHG to 160/195 mmHG (McQueen & Celentano, 1982).

*Pain.* The neurophysiology and biochemistry of pain is one of the six focal dimensions of pain (Karoly, 1985). Traditional assessments of pain using indices such as heart rate, blood pressure, and skin conductance have not proven consistently reliable. A relatively new but promising area is the use of biochemical assays (Terenius, 1980).

*Obesity.* We have already discussed measuring weight and appropriate indices. There are not existing acceptable cutoff points to determine obesity (Bray, 1979). There are varying criteria for the three major indices: power, relative weight, and skin-fold thickness. There is not a clear point at which adverse health effects of being overweight sharply increase, so definitions of obesity are somewhat arbitrary (Stewart et al., 1980).

## SUMMARY

Observation is a direct method for assessing behavior. Observers also have biases, however, and many variables of interest are not observable or are difficult to observe. Systematic observation begins with the creation of categories and systems for observation. The act of observing can affect the behavior being observed, and ways of making observation less intrusive are discussed. Reliability is usually assessed using measures of interobserver agreement. The level of inference involved in the observation is one factor that can influence data validity. Observational measures of cognition and affect are discussed using the example of distress or anxiety. Observational measures of behavior are given for pain behavior and compliance. Observational measures of health status are discussed for pain and functional ability and seizures and other infrequent events.

Physiological measures, while often considered "hard" data, also present problems of reliability and validity. Repeated measures are often needed to improve reliability, and, as with observational measures, the level of inference can affect validity. Physiological measures of cognition and affect are discussed in terms of stress and distress, which exemplify the validity problem. Some common physiological measures of distress include respiration, muscle tension, and catecholamine and corticosteroid secretion. The kinds of arousal that could affect these measures, however, is also dependent on contextual cues. Other completely irrelevant factors can also affect measures of endocrine activity. Examples of physiological measures of behavior are given for smoking, weight control, and substance use. The physiological measurement of health status is the basis of clinical medicine. Some research examples include mortality, morbidity, blood pressure, and obesity. The use of physiological measures in research always requires technical expertise and familiarity with the measures.

## EXERCISES

(1) Devise a system for observing physician/patient interaction. Include verbal as well as nonverbal communication. Then select a television

program that has a medical focus and have two or more observers code physician/patient interactions. Calculate interobserver agreement.

(2) Collect data on the weight and height of 10 people. Compare absolute weights, relative weights, and power indexes. To what extent do these different measures change the rankings of the individuals in the group?

# 9

# *Conducting the Study*

You have chosen your setting, your question, your design, your sample, and your measures. If yours is an experimental study, you have decided what the intervention or manipulation will be, that is, how your experimental group will differ from the control group. You are still far from conducting your study, however. You need to work out your procedures, how the study will actually be conducted, and pilot and refine them. You still have many decisions to make. And then, when the study is finally underway, you still have to be prepared for the unexpected, for threats to validity that suddenly materialize, and for serendipitous events that provide unplanned opportunities. In this chapter, we shall discuss designing an experimental intervention, constructing the interview or questionnaire, developing the procedures, and responding to crises and opportunities as they arise.

## DESIGNING THE INTERVENTION

There are several things to look for when you are translating your construct or idea into your experimental intervention. Most important is consistency of administration. Unless your subjects are actually exposed to the experimental treatment, there will be no test of it. The most dangerous situation is when some situation or event over which you have no control systematically biases exposure. Example 9.1 describes an evaluation of factors that could bias exposure to an intervention in the BSE study.

---

*Example 9.1.*
*Choosing a Reminder System*

In the first BSE study, one of the interventions was to provide a monthly reminder to perform BSE to half the women in the study and compare their compliance rates to the other half of the women who did not receive the reminder (Grady, 1984). We weighed the pros and cons of telephone and mailed reminders to help us decide how to implement the reminder system.

Telephone calls have the advantage of assurance that the target person has been reached and the intervention delivered. They have several disadvantages, however. Repeated efforts may be required to reach the person at home. Lines may be busy. Children and other family members may answer the telephone and not always pass on messages. These difficulties may also be differentially distributed across the population with, for example, younger working women being harder to reach than retired older women. The consistency of exposure to the intervention could thus be biased in systematic ways that we could not control. There is also the very practical problem of the cost in terms of staff time, particularly for evening and weekend calls.

Mailed reminders have the advantage of simplicity of administration. They are easy to prepare and can be sent out in large batches. Exposure could also be biased with a letter, however. People, especially busy people, do not always open their mail right away. The reminder could not function as a reminder unless the participants both received *and* read it. Postcards would answer some of these difficulties but introduce a problem of privacy. A message to the participant about breast self-examination or about being in the study could be read by letter carriers and other family members. We solved this problem by designing the postcard to have only a project "logo" (a hand surrounded by the words "Keep in Touch") on it with no other message. It was also printed on a distinctive yellow card stock as were all project materials, serving as a further reminder of the project. It would stand out in a stack of mail and would have meaning only to the woman herself, as a reminder for BSE.

---

In Example 9.1, we have purposely chosen a very simple translation from a construct ("reminding" or "cuing") to the actual intervention (postcard). More complicated constructs would require much more thought and many more decisions before they were operationalized for the experiment. Other kinds of considerations aside from consistency and ease of administration include respondent burden and ethical issues. In evaluating respondent burden, the health and education of study participants should be considered in relation to the intervention. Is the ability of the subjects to understand and respond to your intervention at all compromised by their health status or level of education? Ethical issues involve potential harm to the participant. (See Chapter 5.) The privacy problem of the postcard reminders for BSE is really an ethical issue. It is important to review your operationalization with many different kinds of people, and particularly ones who are likely to be similar to participants, to see if there are subtle kinds of harm, offensiveness, or cultural insensitivity. Pilot studies, which will be discussed later in this chapter, should test for these kinds of unintended effects.

## Manipulation Checks

It is important to confirm exposure to the intervention/manipulation. This knowledge is particularly critical when you are trying to understand results that differ from your original expectations. Such differences could be because your intervention was not sufficiently powerful, was not remembered, or had a different impact than you expected. A common way to test whether the manipulation worked is to ask simple questions, termed *manipulation checks*, at the *end of the study*. You would expect persons in different conditions to respond differently to the questions. In one of our studies, a standard manipulation check provided a surprising result as described in Example 9.2.

---

*Example 9.2.*
*Checking the Intervention*

In a study about the effects of information and choice of treatment on recovery from surgery, we included several questions on the final interview to check that patients had received the appropriate intervention. We asked separate questions about whether information and choice were provided with the expectation that persons in the choice condition would say yes to both, persons in the information condition would say yes only to information, and persons in the control condition would say no to both. Before asking these questions, we put in a "filler item" that we expected would allow everyone to give a yes response. Because respondents often feel you want them to say yes, it is sometimes helpful to start with a question to which everyone can answer yes. Having said yes once, they might feel freer to say no later. The filler item in this case was a question about whether they had participated in a study. Of our 127 patients, 14 said they had *not* been in a research project during their hospital stay even though they had been visited by our nurses five or six times and all personnel wore large red and white "Health Care Research Project" buttons. This failure to notice any aspect of our study interventions reminded us that in the context of a hospital system where so much goes on, so many people enter patient rooms, and patients are often stressed, manipulations must be powerful to have a long-lasting effect and sometimes even to be noticed.

---

From the manipulation check you may discover that not everyone in the sample was exposed to the manipulation. It is acceptable to test your hypotheses only with the exposed group, but you must carefully note in the research report just how you have selected this subgroup and what biases this selection may introduce into the analysis or interpretation.

For example, in a study of the effects of reward on BSE, the overall finding was that external reward (a lottery ticket or Susan B. Anthony dollar) was superior to both self-reward instruction and a no reward control, which were not different from each other (Grady, Goodenow, & Borkin, in press). An examination of the intervention check, however, showed that only half the participants actually tried self-reward. Analyses on this subgroup showed that those who used self-reward were just be compliant as the external reward group. There are then two conclusions that can be drawn about the efficacy of self-reward in this study: It is only acceptable to about half the women, but, when accepted, it is as effective as external reward. Both conclusions need to be stated to give a complete picture of the effect of this intervention.

## CONSTRUCTING YOUR INSTRUMENTS

Any research project that involves contact with the participants needs a form or "instrument" for data collection. It can be a very simple instrument if there is not much information to gather or it can be lengthy and complex, but the provision of a standard format for data collection will very much simplify administration of the study and later data management and analysis. Even if you are designing a single page for a receptionist to mark appointments kept, and certainly if you are designing anything lengthier, there are some standard pieces of information that should be printed on the form.

*Project I.D.:* The full name of the research project and address should be included.

*Project telephone number:* A telephone number participants can use to call with questions should be provided. This is an ethical as well as data collection issue. People should be given the right (and ability) to ask questions about the project at any time during it. At the same time, participant questions can inform researchers about any problems with data collection.

*I.D. of persons involved in filling out the form:* This identification would involve the interviewer and interviewee, the respondent if it is a questionnaire, or the observer if one is involved.

*Date filled out (including year):* The date is a common omission, but knowing it can be very valuable later on. You think now that you will never forget the year you did the XX project, but it happens. There may also turn out to be some bias in the data that is related to time of year.

*Instructions for filling out form:* These should be as simple as possible while still clear. Do not use more words than you need. Verbosity will stop people from reading the instructions, including the parts they really should know.

## The Interview

There are many good books on interviewing techniques and the construction of the interview (see, for example, Lavrakas, 1987, in this series). If an interview is central to your study, you should refer to a book specifically about this method. Here we will review some of the basic elements of the interview to provide a framework within which to make decisions during the construction of the interview.

An interview is a structured conversation. When the interviewer and the interviewee sit down together to have this structured conversation, it is basically a social situation. All the usual social amenities apply. When the interview instrument is being developed, this social situation should be kept in mind. The interview should be developed to maintain as much naturalness as possible. What follows are some tips to maintain a conversational atmosphere.

*(1) Introduce yourself and explain what you are going to do.* Your structured conversation might open like this: "Hello, Mrs. Jones. I'm Sally Smith with the Health Care Research Project. We have some questions about your health, how you feel about the health care you are getting, and some questions about your background. The whole interview should take about 20 minutes."

*(2) Start where they are.* Try to imagine what the respondent might be thinking at the start of the interview. Why are they where they are (in a hospital bed, in a doctor's office, at home on the telephone with you)? What else is going on? What do they already know about the study? You might begin with a question like, "Why did you decide to be in the study?" If the respondent is a patient and you have some health-status questions, you might start with them: "How do you feel today?" "How long have you had (the condition)?" *Do not* start with embarrassing or difficult questions or with ones with a complicated response format. Questions on age, income, and religion are often refused by respondents. If you ask them too early, you run the risk of having the interview terminated. If they are placed at the end of the interview, termination is less of a problem.

*(3) Phrase your questions in plain English.* Try not to use multisyllabic words and technical terms. A word like *responsibility* may seem

common enough but it is a six-syllable word. The phrase *up to you* can convey the same meaning as "your responsibility." If you have to use technical terms, explain them. For example, "Do you have a primary care physician, by that I mean a doctor you see for all your regular health care needs, checkups, colds, and so forth?"

*(4) Flow from one topic to another.* Organize the elements of your interview by topic, for example, put the health-status scales with the other health questions. Then organize the topics so that there is a flow from one to the other. Transitions will still be necessary, for example, "And now I'd like to ask you some questions about . . .." When writing the transitions for the interviewer, avoid long speeches. Again, think about a conversation. Ideally, you would like the respondent talking more than the interviewer. People also can't listen and understand long, overrehearsed speeches that are read to them. Memorized speeches tend to sound rote because inflection is missing or is oddly placed.

*(5) Pay attention to your response format.* How you word the questions is obviously important, but how you word the answers (i.e., the response format) can be equally important. Some of your questions will have a scale for an answer. For established instruments, you will probably be using whatever scale the developers created. (See Chapter 7, on self-reports, for when and how to modify existing scales.) Within topics, group together similar response formats to minimize the amount of instruction needed. If you are creating some of your own scaled items, you can choose a response format similar to the scale immediately preceding or following it or you can choose your own scale. Some scales will be more familiar to your respondents than others. For example, a "0 to 10" scale may be easier for a respondent than a scale of "1 to 7." If you have a 3-point scale, just use the words (e.g., "never," "sometimes," "always") and omit the numbers.

*(6) Use a response card.* If your scale is complicated, with unfamiliar categories or many labeled scale points, provide a written version of the possible responses, a response card, which can be handed to the respondent. You cannot expect respondents to remember a lot of categories or what the number "5" is supposed to mean. It is a good idea also to use a response card when asking potentially embarrassing questions, such as income. With your income categories printed on the card and identified by letters, the interviewer can hand it to the respondent and say, "Just indicate which letter comes closest to your present family income." Even with a response card, the interviewer should read the categories. Remember, not everyone can read and some people have vision problems.

*(7) Do not use needless categories.* Sometimes categories help, as with the income question, and sometimes they just add complexity to the interview. Whenever possible, taking a number as a response is better than creating groups of numbers. For example, for the question, "How many BSEs have you done in the last year?," simply take the number as a response rather than create categories like "none," "some," "a few," or categories like "0-3," "4-6," and so on. It will save interview time not to have to read the categories and will also provide more flexibility in your data analysis.

*(8) Use open-ended questions for transitions, exploration, or elaboration.* Sometimes a question will elicit a difficult or painful admission, such as the respondent has had cancer or that a close family member recently died. It is socially awkward and somewhat insensitive to record that fact and then press on with the rest of the interview. An open-ended question can give the respondent an opportunity to comment on the event and make transition to the next topic easier. Open-ended questions can also be used for exploration when you really do not know what the response categories should be. You are, therefore, forced to leave the question open-ended. Open-ended questions used for elaboration can be valuable for understanding a phenomenon more fully, providing richness to the data while conveying to the respondent that you really are interested in her or his experiences and not just numbers.

*(9) Thank them at the end.* You should always thank the respondents. They are doing you a favor. Without the willingness of respondents to answer questions, there would be no social or behavioral research. End the interview on a positive, up-beat note, assuring them that they have been very helpful and that you are grateful.

## The Questionnaire

A questionnaire or survey is a facsimile of an interview. During its construction, the implied social situation must be kept in mind. Like the interview, the questionnaire should start where the respondent is, make sense, and flow like a structured conversation. You should avoid lengthy directions and explanations. Minimal directions should be used because there is a very good chance that they will not be read. Headings can be used to set off topics rather than the sentence that would be used in an interview; for example, "Health Questions" can replace "And now I'd like to ask you some questions about your health."

The response format suggestions offered for the interview also apply with minor modifications to the questionnaire. Group questions and scales by topic and within topic by response format. Some common sense needs to be applied: Scale questions that go on for more than a page can become boring and respondents can adopt a "response set" of always agreeing or disagreeing. The layout should be visually interesting so that it holds attention and should be clearly marked into sections so that progress can be felt.

The social etiquette requirements for a questionnaire are not as stringent as for an interview. Open-ended questions do not need to be provided for transition or elaboration because space for comments can be left at the end. You need only include open-ended questions for exploration, that is, when you have no idea what the response categories might be. It is still important to thank respondents at the end of the questionnaire. For more detailed information, see Fowler (1984, in this series).

## DEVELOPING THE PROCEDURES

There are numerous decisions to be made about exactly how to proceed with the research, how to put it all together. Considerations involve who should handle each piece and when and where various things should be done.

### Who

Who should administer measures in your studies? Who should be involved in the intervention? There may be restrictions in health care settings that you need to attend to as you consider this. In some circumstances, it is important to have trained personnel, such as nurses, do the manipulations or be available should there be any health care issues. For example, in the surgery study, the manipulations involving choices and information were always administered by RNs. They had the appropriate knowledge to interact with patients on patient care issues. Their involvement also added external validity given that adoption of these procedures in a hospital would likely be a nursing function. Because of the control we wished to have, we chose to use nurses on our staff rather than hospital nurses. Consequently, only a few nurses were involved and training was minimized. The research wasn't a task squeezed into a busy service function; it was *the* task for our nurses. Under other circumstances, existing hospital staff may be a more convenient and economical choice. In either case, some involvement of existing staff in the project and training is critical, as discussed in Chapter 2.

In deciding who shall collect data, research and practical considerations may conflict. It is important, if at all possible, for persons collecting dependent measures to be unaware of experimental conditions because experimenters can subtly influence the outcome of studies (Rosenthal, 1976). (Traditionally, this has been known as being "blind" to the condition, but because that language can be offensive, we shall use the more neutral "lack of awareness" of condition.) Thus, in the surgical study, we decided that data on the patients should be collected by people other than the RNs who administered the interventions. Because patient care was not involved, we were able to use graduate students in these roles. In fact, because of things patients said, lack of awareness was not always complete, but, among project personnel, information on the condition was not exchanged. It might have been more economical to use the same persons in both roles but separating the roles was preferable from the research standpoint. In Example 9.3, a way of using the same person in both roles is described.

---

*Example 9.3.*
*Controlling Experimenter Bias*

In the BSE studies, the procedure called for both teaching BSE, usually a clinical function, and interviewing and explaining experimental procedures, tasks usually best done by someone with research training. The decision was made to hire research assistants and train them as lay BSE instructors rather than hire people with clinical experience and try to teach them all the subtle ways the results might be biased by their actions. The problem still remained that knowing the experimental condition of the women might affect the way BSE was taught. It was crucial that the method of teaching and the resulting competence in BSE be held as constant as possible across conditions. Knowing that someone was assigned to the control condition, for example, might make the teaching more thorough because the research assistant knew these women would be receiving no extra help throughout the project, or it might make the teaching less thorough because the research assistant accepted the hypothesis that these women would be less compliant. A procedure was, therefore, developed to keep the research assistant unaware of experimental condition until *after* the teaching. All project materials, including those relevant to the experimental condition, were placed in separate envelopes for each participant and identification numbers were randomly assigned to the conditions. During the teaching, the research assistant knew the identification number but was unaware of the condition assignment. After the teaching, if the woman agreed to be in the study, the envelope was opened, the condition revealed, and appropriate study instructions were given. This procedure also ensured that the request to be in the project was not made more or less enthusiastically depending on the experimental condition.

## When and Where

Should data collection be postsurgery or presurgery or both? Should telephone calls be made early in the morning or in the evening? Should the weight loss programs be scheduled for the summer or winter? Should data collection be part of the clinical visit or separate? Some decisions about when procedures should take place will be dictated by the experimental design or question. Others will be constrained by practical considerations. It is still worthwhile to review the implications of these decisions. Time in the course of treatment, time of day, and seasonal variations can affect who participates in your study as well as the degree of cooperation. What happens in the clinical visit can affect the ability or motivation of your participants. If it seems that some aspect of timing might affect your data and you cannot revise your procedures to rule out that effect, you may want to include that timing factor as a variable in your study and record it for each participant. If time is constant across participants, you may consider its effects in discussing results and considering generalizability. Kelly and McGrath (1988), in this series, provide an in-depth discussion of the role of time and timing in research.

Where should the procedures take place? Should the interview be conducted at work or at home or wherever the participant can be reached? Should the health education be conducted in a clinical setting or a nonclinical setting? Is there anything about the setting that is likely to raise the blood pressure of the participant when blood pressure is one of your key measures? Is there anything about the setting that is likely to make participants particularly comfortable or uncomfortable? In short, is there anything about the setting that is likely to affect the motivation, ability, or health status of your participants? Again, if you think there is and you cannot correct the problem, you will want to include variations in setting as a variable or note the limitations the setting imposes on your conclusions.

## How

There are numerous choices to be made about exactly how to proceed, and many decisions will be study-specific. Some common questions concern how to choose between an interview and a question-naire and how to increase responses to mailed questionnaires. There are some general considerations when making these decisions.

An interview is much more expensive than a questionnaire when staff time is taken into account. Questionnaires are easier and cheaper to administer, but the quality of the data is generally much poorer than from an interview. Respondents are more likely to skip questions (or even whole pages) and to misread or misunderstand directions. Responses to exploratory open-ended questions are often better recorded by an interviewer. Questions with a complicated response format or sequence (e.g., "If yes on question #24, answer questions #25 a-f; If no, skip to question #26") are sometimes better given by a trained interviewer. On the other hand, questions with a very simple response format (e.g., true-false personality inventories) are often easier in a questionnaire than an interview. The issues of expense and the quality and kind of data needed should be weighed in terms of the particular requirements of the study.

Sometimes interviews and questionnaires can be combined to collect different types of data. For example, in a one-year follow-up in a BSE study, a questionnaire was sent to collect attitude and stressful life event data. Responses to the attitude items involved circling numbers on Likert-type scales, a task easier done with the scales and their categories presented visually. The stressful life event measure involved simply checking which of 103 events had happened to the participant in the last year. Reading all of these items aloud would have taken a long time in an interview. The mailed questionnaire was followed up by a telephone interview to collect more qualitative and exploratory data about participants' reactions to the study and information about any breast changes found. Thus the methods were matched to the types of data needed in an effort to obtain high-quality data of both types.

There are some standard ways for increasing responses to mailed questionnaires. (A good source of tips for conducting mail and telephone surveys is a book by Dillman, 1978, and, in this series, one by Fowler, 1984.) First of all, the questionnaire should look as *simple* to do as possible. Brevity is a good idea but format is at least as important. The typeface should be legible, and the layout, interesting and clear. Returning the questionnaire should be facilitated by provision of a stamped preaddressed envelope. Second, a *token of appreciation* can be included. One of us once filled out an eight-page questionnaire on cultural life in Springfield, Massachusetts, simply because attached to the cover letter was a quarter to be used "to brighten the day of a child you know." In one of the BSE studies, the final questionnaire (the one least likely to be returned) was sent with a crisp one-dollar bill as "a very small return for the information you have generously provided." In a rheumatoid arthritis study, a pencil was enclosed both as a material token and a means of making filling out the questionnaire easier.

The *cover letter* is also important. It should be on letterhead, preferably institutional letterhead with a logo, but you can make up letterhead for your project, for example, "The Health Care Research Project," with an address. It should look as much like a personal letter as possible rather than like a form letter. The cover letter should be short (certainly no more than one page) and include the following elements: a brief description of the purposes of the project, how important it is for that person to respond, how participants were selected, and how to get further information about the project. The purpose is to solicit their participation and to give them some sense of why their particular participation is valuable.

The most important way to increase response, however, is through *follow-up*. It is generally estimated that each follow-up contact elicits half as many responses as the previous one. About one week after the questionnaire goes out, send a postcard to everyone with a message like "Thank you for your help and if you haven't mailed back the questionnaire, please do." Because only one week has elapsed, nonrespondents will not yet feel guilty and may happily respond at that time, and respondents will be thanked. About three weeks later, we recommend another contact to nonrespondents only. This can be a letter or a postcard, again requesting their help and offering to answer any questions. Three weeks later, a final, stronger letter can be sent reiterating most of the points of the first letter and including another copy of the questionnaire. To some extent, the number of follow-up contacts appropriate for your study can be determined by how successful each contact is in eliciting further responses.

## Pilot Studies

After you have made decisions about who, when, where, and how your study procedures are going to be implemented, you should check each aspect of your procedure to uncover any flaws or oversights. Start with yourself and your study team by role-playing. For example, administer the interview to each other, checking for timing and transitions. Try answering the questions honestly, as yourself, and then as participants with different kinds of histories, particularly problematic ones such as significant health problems. You may find questions that need to be reworded, response formats that need to be changed, transitions that need to be added, or important omissions that need to be corrected. After corrections are made, role-play the new version.

All aspects of the study should be checked. In the BSE studies where participants were individually taught how to do a breast self-examination, the teaching was rehearsed many times. This rehearsal not only pinpointed problems but gave the three teachers an opportunity to learn the teaching protocol and match their teaching styles.

Increasing realism should be introduced into these role-plays. The adequacy of the planned setting should be checked. In the above examples, the interview should be administered in the place it will be given and the teaching should be rehearsed where it is going to be done. Noise and other distractions, lack of privacy, even room temperature may affect your planned procedures.

When from a research perspective you are satisfied with your procedures, small pilot studies should be done. Pilot participants should be recruited who are as similar to the expected study participants as possible. After the pilot participants have gone through your procedure, discuss their reactions in depth. You can then learn whether your measures are understandable, whether your manipulations are having the expected effect, whether there are any offensive aspects, and where there are other flaws. Because pilot work is not a formal study and is typically not reported, you may make procedural changes as you go along. Once an actual study is started, procedures should not be changed.

## AS THE STUDY GOES ALONG

Many things can happen during the course of the study that have the potential for influencing the results. This influence can be positive or negative and, from a research perspective, hardly matters. The direction of influence is not as important as the possibility that there will be no meaningful results because of some unforeseen event. Reacting to the problem can take many forms. You can merely note the problem in your research report, in either the method section or the interpretation of results. You can change your procedures and discard previously collected data. You can add a variable and analyze your results taking into account this new variable that reflects the problem. You can collect additional data. In this section, we shall consider three examples of problems that can occur as the study goes along and that require different coping strategies.

## Changes in Public Awareness

The extensive media coverage of President Reagan's diagnosis of colon cancer in July 1985 undoubtedly raised public awareness of colon cancer and perhaps even cancer in general. Similar sudden increases in public awareness were caused in the 1970s by the breast cancer diagnoses of Betty Ford and Happy Rockefeller. In both cases, clinicians reported sudden increases in the number of patients requesting cancer screening. Anyone who had a study underway that involved knowledge of cancer, attitudes related to cancer, or cancer screening behavior faced a likely change in participants' data before and after these major media events.

Some changes in public awareness are more gradual or occur in a more scattered manner. A particular magazine may feature an article on a disease or condition that you are studying. Only the readers of that magazine would then be affected. Similarly, a television show may be broadcast with the potential to contaminate your study but only for the people who saw or heard about it. Scattered reports about herpes, for example, have raised public awareness somewhat, but awareness may be most acute among single people who are dating.

What can one do to control the threat to validity that such changes in public awareness cause? There are several steps that can be taken. If every instance of data collection has been dated (as it should be), then data before and after a specific consciousness-raising event can be clearly identified. Responses can be compared to determine whether there are differences attributable to the event. Study hypotheses may still be able to be tested within these differences. For a more sensitive assessment of the impact of either a specific event or gradual shifts in awareness, additional questions may be devised to ask each participant about awareness. Responses to these questions then provide additional predictor variables in the study. If there is a possibility that awareness may vary by sociodemographic characteristics as in the herpes example, this can be directly tested and any resulting interactions can become predictors.

## Unexpectedly Poor Data

Even though you spent a lot of time reviewing the procedures for data collection and conducting pilot tests, when the study is actually fielded, the initial data may be inadequate. In Chapter 2, "Health Care Settings and Collaborative Research," the example was given of the dental study where the first batches of data were incomplete and ratings were remarkably similar across patients. The problem was that the dental hygienists, who were collecting the data, had not been included in the decision-making process and did not appreciate data collection requirements. Piloting in that case should have included not only a sample of patients similar to the proposed subjects but a sample of dental hygienists similar to those who would be collecting the data. In the end, the inadequate data had to be treated as a pilot and discarded.

## Too Few Subjects

In Chapter 5, "Selecting the Sample," we discussed the problem of "chasing every case." Reasonable estimates of how many participants can be recruited may be made during the planning stages of the research, but when recruitment is actually underway, it may become clear that the target goal will not be achieved. If you cannot make do with fewer subjects, more aggressive recruiting procedures have to be considered or the addition of another data collection site. In either case, the necessary changes yield new variables that must be included in the data analysis. When considering a change in site, the characteristics of the additional site must be carefully weighed as we discussed in Chapter 2. Comparability of data from two sites cannot be assumed without evaluating any potential differences. It is particularly important that ways in which the sample might differ be included as variables in the study.

## SUMMARY

Before a study can actually be conducted, there are many decisions to be made about procedures. If it is an experimental study, the manipulation needs to be designed, taking into account ease and consistency of administration, respondent burden, and ethical considerations. Manipulation checks should be included at the end of the study. In most studies, data collection instruments need to be devised and should include standard identifying information and clear instructions for completion. An interview, which is a structured conversation, needs to be designed keeping in mind the social amenities. Questionnaires are facsimiles of interviews and many of the same guidelines apply. In developing procedures, consideration must be given to who should administer measures, when and where data should be collected, and how choices should be made about an interview versus a questionnaire. If a mailed questionnaire is chosen, there are things you can do to increase the response rate. Pilot studies should always be undertaken to check all aspects of the procedure. As the study goes along, unforeseen events occur requiring procedural adjustments or additions.

## EXERCISES

(1) Develop a short interview about health status and health care. Collect background information (i.e., age, sex, race, educational level, marital status, employment status) as well. Structure both the questions and the possible responses.

(2) Pilot your interview on two to three people who are likely to differ on health status. Are there questions that are unclear or responses you did not anticipate? Revise the interview accordingly.

# 10

## *Interpreting and Publishing Findings*

For many researchers, interpreting and publishing the results of the study are the hardest tasks in research. There is hardly a researcher who does not have unpublished results, either because interpretation was difficult or because the initial report was rejected for publication. What starts out as a simple hypothesis can become complicated in the execution and explanation. Then, too, many people have blocks about statistics or about writing. Feeling insecure about our abilities, we can procrastinate forever. In this chapter, we shall touch on the subjects of analyzing your data, making inferences from the results, and communicating your findings with a view toward helping you past some of the common pitfalls.

### DATA ANALYSIS

You have collected your data and you need to understand what you now know. For many people, this is a difficult part because *statistics* are involved. It is important and healthy to put statistics in their place. They are only tools. They can help you compile and organize your data. They can help you assess what you really know. They can also help you tell your story. In some sciences, statistics are not used because anyone looking at the data can clearly get the picture. Graphing the data from time-series and single-subject designs (Chapter 4) can often present a powerful visual argument for the effects of an intervention. Statistics might make us more confident of these effects, but they are often not necessary. For most of our research, however, the findings are not so clear-cut and statistics can help us a great deal.

#### Getting Help

If you are not familiar with data analysis, you will need some assistance. There are a few written sources of help that we recommend.

In a very brief chapter (20 pages), Wagenaar (1981) provides a review of social science statistics without formulas. You will not be able to conduct analyses after reading this chapter, but it can be very helpful in conjunction with a statistical consultant. It is likely to enable you to understand the consultant better.

At a more sophisticated level, but designed to be readable by someone with one undergraduate course in statistics, is Tabachnick and Fidell's (1983) volume on multivariate statistics. They focus on the use and interpretation of statistics in an attempt to answer the questions important to researchers: "Which analytic technique is most useful for answering my research question?" "How do my data fit the technique?" "How do I interpret the results in terms of the research question?" (p. xv). They also provide examples of results sections in journal format for each statistic.

Linton and Gallo's (1975) is a practical guide to correct data analysis. They provide step-by-step computation with examples and interpretation. They cover nonparametric and parametric techniques. Statistics books all use different nomenclature so it may be best to stay with the text you are used to and on which you were trained.

If you have not had formal training in statistics or do not feel confident of your own abilities, you may also want to use a statistical consultant. In addition to involving a consultant early in the study, it is important to select one carefully. You want someone who is familiar with the type of data you have. There are different statistical traditions. Biostatisticians tend to use correlational/regression approaches. Psychological statisticians are more likely to use analysis of variance as a primary framework. While regression and analysis of variance are statistically comparable, the language of communication and the nature of understanding may be quite different. If you are more comfortable with the language of one or the other of these approaches, try to find a consultant who comes from a similar tradition.

It is important to be able to communicate with your statistical consultant. If the consultant constantly is talking at a level beyond your understanding, *you* are *not* at fault, except in having selected the wrong consultant. You must be assertive and ask questions whenever you do not understand something. Your consultant should bring you closer to rather than distance you from your data. The consultant should be willing to take what you know and deliver findings back to you in a form you can understand. We observed a statistical consultant provide a long, involved discourse on data analysis. At the conclusion, the researcher still had to ask her question, "But did the participants lose any weight?"

## Choosing Statistics

The step of planning your analyses really comes *before* you have collected your data. Analysis issues are important as they are related to sample size (see Chapter 5). They may also alert you to measures that you need to collect. Linton and Gallo (1975) and Tabachnick and Fidell (1983) provide decision trees to help select a statistic.

You begin with your question. If you have more than one question, you may need to employ several statistics. Is your question about differences, about degrees of relationship between variables, or an attempt to predict group membership? For example, the question in the arthritis learned helplessness study is about the degree of relationship between arthritis severity and helplessness. This requires a measure of association. The question in the surgical study is about differences between groups that were treated differently (information, choice, and control). Some form of testing significance of the difference between groups is needed. In the BSE studies, when we compared nonparticipants to participants (Grady et al., 1983), we were trying to predict group membership. Discriminant function analysis is the appropriate statistic.

## Preliminary Analyses

Before you move on to conducting the major statistical test of your hypothesis, it is necessary to start with descriptive statistics. Descriptive statistics describe your sample in terms of the variables measured. They are important in your presentation of results in order to give the reader a more complete picture of the bases of your conclusions. You need to be sure that your data are "clean"—that there are no errors. Statistics that describe the nature of your data help in the detection of errors. For example, if each item on your scale has a potential range of 1 to 6, an 8 must be in error. Look at the minimum, maximum, and mean and standard deviations in search of such out-of-range values. You should have some idea of expected overall means for your measures. Numbers that are very out of line may imply an error. You also need to assess the distribution of the variables to see that they meet the assumptions of your statistical tests. Departures from normality may require transformation of variables (see Tabachnick & Fidell, 1983). Very large standard deviations may imply *outliers*, that is, extreme scores that may disproportionally affect your statistics.

Preliminary analyses should also be used to test for extraneous differences between groups. When an extra site has been used to increase the sample size and differences between the sites are not wanted or expected, preliminary analyses should be conducted to check for differences. If there are differences, the data cannot be combined and the site should become a variable in analyses. If there are other unanticipated differences between groups on a variable that may be related to your dependent measure, there are statistical techniques for controlling for or *covarying* out the effects of such variables. For example, even though we had randomly assigned patients to condition in one of our studies, patients in the three conditions differed in education. Therefore, we used education as a covariate for all analyses (Wallston et al., 1987).

Once you have done these initial data analyses, you need to consider a series of issues in selecting the major statistic to test your hypothesis. As you do analyses, continue to look for anomalies in your computer printout. While computers don't make mistakes, researchers do. If your analyses do not make sense, check *very carefully* in search of errors.

## Number of Variables

To choose your statistics, you always need to know the number of independent (or predictor) variables and the number of dependent (or criterion) variables. One of each requires a *bivariate* statistic. When you have more than one independent or dependent variable, a *multivariate* analysis is appropriate.

## Level of Measurement

The level of measurement of your variables also determines the appropriate statistics. For *nominal* data, numbers are arbitrarily assigned to categories because there are no numerical values. Examples of nominal variables are sex, religion, and the presence or absence of a disease. *Ordinal* data are ranked. For example, to measure health value, we ask people to rank 10 values in order of importance. We know that the value ranked first is most important, but we cannot tell how close or far it is from the value ranked second. *Interval* data specifies the order and that the distance between numbers (the intervals) are equal. IQ is an example of interval data. Likert scales (e.g., agree–disagree using a scale of 1-5) are usually treated as interval data although the equality of the intervals is debatable. *Ratio* data have a real 0, and we can say that a person 50 years old is twice as old as someone who is 25. *Nonparametric* statistics must be used for nominal and ordinal data while *parametric* statistics are used for interval and ratio data.

## Measures of Association

The bivariate measure of association is a correlation (*r*). For parametric data, a *Pearson's r* is used. For ordinal data, *Spearman's rho* is the most commonly used measure. For nominal data, there are a number of measures including *phi* and *Goodman and Kruskal's tau.* Correlations can range from -1 to +1. They assess the strength and direction of relation. Statistical tests are used to assess the probability that a correlation is reliably different from 0.

With multiple predictors, a *regression* allows the detection of the degree of association. A combination of independent variables is created to predict to the criterion best. The multiple correlation (R) when it is squared tells the amount of variance in the criterion associated with the set of predictors. When there are multiple dependent and independent variables, a *canonical correlation* assesses the optimum association between a linear combination of each.

## Measures of Difference

Again, you must make the nonparametric/parametric distinction. For nonparametric data, Siegel (1956) has a table on the inside cover to assist in selecting appropriate nonparametric statistics. The most common test is *chi-square*. Differences between groups on a single dependent measure can be assessed using chi-square. With more than one independent variable, you can partition chi-square to create main and interaction effects analogous to analysis of variance (Linton & Gallo, 1975).

With parametric data, a single independent variable with only two levels and a single dependent variable, the *t-test* is used. For multiple independent variables or a single variable with more than two levels, *analysis of variance* is used. For analysis of variance, the independent variables need only be nominal (as in the three treatment conditions of the surgical example). A variable that is interval can be broken into categories to use analysis of variance. If you wish to use the full range of that variable, *regression* would be the appropriate statistic. Thus the distinction between group differences and measures of association may become fuzzy. With multiple independent and dependent variables, *multivariate analysis of variance* is used.

## Predicting Group Membership

When the dependent measure or criterion is nominal, *discriminant function analysis,* which parallels regression, is used. For example, in the arthritis study, in addition to the regressions discussed, we plan to select a group of people who appear to be doing really well and another group who appear helpless. A discriminant function analysis will allow us to ascertain the combination of independent variables that will discriminate between these groups.

## MAKING INFERENCES

Having done your data analyses, you need to figure out what you know. The first question is whether your hypothesis or model was confirmed. If the answer is yes, and the results are clear-cut with no effects you did not foresee, then you can move to writing. This is, however, a rare occurrence in science. Usually something unexpected has occurred and untangling the meaning can be an interesting and creative task. If your findings do not confirm your hypothesis, your goal is to understand what you have found. When the results are messy, you will typically want to attempt further analysis until you understand your data.

If your study was an experiment, the first place to look is at the *manipulation* check. Did the manipulation work? If it did not, you may need to do another study with a stronger manipulation. If it worked for some people, however, you can first attempt an internal analysis, looking at data for only those people who correctly answered the manipulation check. You no longer have a randomized experiment because you are violating random assignment, and you have less power because subjects are being eliminated; but if you get the results you expected for subjects for whom the manipulation worked, it provides some confidence in your hypothesis. You may also want to examine differences between subjects for whom the manipulation worked, and those for whom it did not work. It may be that your hypothesis needs to be expanded into an interaction that includes an individual difference variable, such as age or health status.

If the manipulation check does not solve your problem, you need to search for any other major confounding variables. Was there a particular doctor or experimenter that had some effect? Did effect vary depending on sex, employment status, or some other demographic variable? If your study was correlational, the predicted association may also be found within such nominal demographic variables. Whatever subsequent analyses you try, note that additional analyses should *not* be purely a fishing expedition. You should have some hypothesis or logical explanation for everything you try.

What about findings you just cannot explain? This depends on how important they are in the context of your results. A single unexplainable three-way interaction in the midst of a series of reasonable results can be mentioned and passed over. A major result you cannot explain requires further thinking and probably another study. In thinking about your results and what they mean, you need to go beyond tests of statistical significance. These tests merely imply that the results are not likely to be due to chance. They should not be confused with the lay use of the word *significance* to mean importance. *Practical significance* or importance is related to the size of the effect (Wallston & Grady, 1985). In this series, see Rosenthal (1984) for methods for interpreting small size effects. You may find a reliable difference between groups equivalent to a tenth of a point on a 10-point scale. Or you may reliably predict 1% of the variance in your criterion. These findings may be of interest theoretically, but their clinical or practical significance is quite limited. You are unlikely to recommend policy changes in the health field based on such small effects. The clinical significance of effect size, however, also depends on the nature of the variables used (Yeaton & Sechrest, 1981). If you can reliably reduce deaths 1% of the time with an inexpensive treatment, this finding can have practical importance if a large number of people die of the disease in question.

In making inferences from your data, you also need to consider any limitations of your study. How is the sample biased (see Chapter 5)? Can you make a case for *external validity* or the generalizability of your findings to other samples, other settings, and other times? Consider again all the threats to validity discussed in Chapter 4. Do you need to do further analyses to show that control groups are equivalent or to rule out other alternative explanations? You want to discuss your data in their best light but also to recognize and discuss their limitations.

## COMMUNICATING YOUR FINDINGS

You have decided what your findings mean and you want to write about them. Before you formally write up your study, you need to determine your audience. Whom do you want to tell? Will these results be most interesting and important to health practitioners, to social and behavioral scientists, to health scientists, to people interested in a particular disease, to policymakers, or to the general public? The outlet you choose, typically a journal, is geared to a particular audience, and the story you tell has to be directed to that audience. There are ethical constraints against multiple publication of the same results in scientific journals. You may, however, be able to rewrite your story for consumers, practitioners, or policymakers without violating this rule.

Publication is not the only way to communicate your findings. Presentation to colleagues is a valuable method for obtaining feedback on the study, especially the conclusions and implications of your work. Such presentations include "brown-bag" seminars, colloquia, poster and paper sessions, or symposia at scientific meetings. You should seek out such opportunities to discuss your study prior to publication as a less formal way to receive feedback.

### Authorship Credit

Who are the authors of the paper and in what order? Disciplines and professions differ in the way this decision is handled. Different research team members may have different experiences and consequently different expectations about authorship. Conflict about publication credit is not uncommon. Decisions about authorship should be discussed as early as possible in the collaborative arrangement. Making such decisions early or at least establishing some rules by which they will be made can reduce later conflict. Where several publications are likely to result from the same research project, these can best be discussed collectively and in advance of data collection.

The American Psychological Association (1983) suggests *substantial scientific contribution* as the guiding principle for the assignment of publication credit. Such contributions include formulating the problem or hypothesis, structuring the experimental design, organizing and conducting the statistical analysis, interpreting the results, or writing a major portion of the paper. Authors should be listed in decreasing order of contribution. Lesser contributions, which do not constitute authorship, include such supportive functions as designing or building the apparatus, suggesting or advising about the statistical analysis, collecting the data, modifying or structuring a computer program, arranging for research subjects, and clerical or similar nonprofessional assistance. Such contributions should be acknowledged in a footnote.

Some researchers use a "rule of thumb" that whoever writes the first draft is the first author on that paper. Such a rule is open to abuse. There is no substitute for having a group discussion and decision about writing and authorship. In no case should a paper be written and submitted without consulting the other professional members of the research team. Although omission of an author is a common cause for conflict, inclusion of someone's name without permission is also a problem. All authors should have an opportunity to read and edit any paper submitted with their names on it.

### Choosing an Outlet

When you have some idea of your desired audience, you should skim potential journals to see where your work will most likely fit. Consider first those journals that have published articles that have served as the foundation of your research. If none of these is appropriate, you may undertake a more general search. A helpful resource is the *Author's Guide to Journals in the Health Field* (Ardell & James, 1980). Swencionis (1982) compiled a list of 48 journals publishing material relevant to health psychology. New journals are constantly being established, however, so archival listings of journals are usually somewhat out of date. Another approach is to search by author using the *Social Science Citation Index*. You can see in what journals researchers doing similar work are cited. It is also helpful to talk to people in the appropriate field.

Within most groups of journals, there are hierarchies. If you believe your work is outstanding, you want to submit it to the best possible outlet with the appropriate audience. More modest contributions may require a less prestigious outlet, but you may still wish to "shoot high" and give yourself the advantage of the excellent critique that you may receive from a top journal even though the manuscript is rejected. You may develop your own hierarchy of submission in advance, realistically anticipating rejection.

The more general the outlet, the more difficult is publication. For example, the *Journal of the American Medical Association* and the *American Psychologist,* which is the primary journal of the American Psychological Association, reach broad audiences of physicians and psychologists. Because articles must have broad appeal, their rejection rates are liable to be quite high. In contrast, the more restricted and specific the outlet, the easier it is to publish appropriate material, because a lesser contribution will still be of interest to experts in the field. Health research must have broader ramifications to be published in a journal whose focus is broader than health. Some journals have a theoretical focus. Others are more interested in applications. You need to be aware of these distinctions.

Most journals have some criteria in common. Most will use two or three reviewers to help evaluate the importance of the research question and findings from the perspective of the readership or mission of the journal. They will assess the method for design flaws. They will also evaluate the clarity of writing. Eichorn and VandenBos (1985) provide a helpful overview on publishing in American Psychological Association journals.

Journals all provide statements as to the kinds of material that are of interest. Often these are found in the inside front cover or on the first couple of pages. For example, the *Journal of Behavioral Medicine* describes itself as

> a broadly conceived interdisciplinary publication devoted to furthering our understanding of physical health and illness through the knowledge and techniques of behavioral science. Application of this knowledge to prevention, treatment and rehabilitation is also a major function of the journal. Typical research areas of interest include: the study of appetitive disorders (alcoholism, smoking, obesity) that serve as physical risk factors, adherence to medical regimen, and health maintenance behavior; pain; self-regulation therapies and biofeedback for somatic disorders; sociocultural influences on health and illness; and brain-behavioral relationships that influence physiological function.

*Research in Nursing and Health* "invites research reports on nursing practice, education, and administration, on health issues relevant to

nursing, and on applications of research findings in clinical settings."
Note that the same research might be published in both journals, but the
orientation of the article—the story you try to tell—would be different.

Examination of the names of the editors and the editorial board is
also helpful. You can see whether there are people in your field and
people who are doing work related to yours represented on the board.
That will give you some idea of the kind of judgments you are likely to
encounter during the review process. The policy statement for *Health
Psychology* sounds quite parallel to that of the *Journal of Behavioral
Medicine*. It even states that "the readership has a broad range of
backgrounds, interests and specializations often interdisciplinary in
nature." Perusal of the editorial boards, however, shows that manuscripts will be reviewed by psychologists. *Behavioral Medicine*, in
contrast, has M.D.s and Ph.D.s from a number of fields represented on
its board. The reviews obtained are likely to be quite different.

## Writing and Submitting Your Work

Once you have selected a journal for your initial submission, you
should review their instructions. Journals vary in referencing format
and other stylistic considerations. It is important to write in the style
appropriate to the journal of interest. Discussing how to write an article
is beyond our scope. A helpful chapter on writing the research report
was prepared by Daryl Bem (1981, 1986).

Before submitting your manuscript, have a colleague unfamiliar with
the project informally evaluate it (and remember to acknowledge their
assistance in a footnote). Because we are so close to our work, it is easy
to omit details and assume the reader will understand. When possible,
get feedback from people familiar with the journal you have chosen.

Once you have submitted the manuscript, go on to other things. It is
going to be several months before you get feedback. When you do get
the letter from the editor, be prepared for rejection. It is the most likely
result. But *do not give up!* There are different kinds of rejection. Many
letters will ask you to revise and resubmit. This is a very positive sign and
you should certainly pursue it. Even outright rejection letters may
suggest alternative journal outlets that are more appropriate. Also,
reviews should provide help in revising, and your revised manuscript is
likely to be of interest to another journal.

Try to be objective about the review you receive and don't take it
personally. Most reviewers are not identified to authors and often

authors are not identified to the reviewers. This procedure, called "blind review," provides a shield of anonymity that sometimes allows people to be unnecessarily cruel. Remember that a review is only one person's opinion. Have someone else look it over to assist you in considering the review. Often you will get helpful feedback from careful reading of a review. Editors make final decisions, and diplomatic negotiations are possible in those cases where reviewers were used inappropriately for either the content or the method of your study.

Most manuscripts can be published with sufficient persistence. Wallston's (1973) manuscript on maternal employment was rejected by four journals before it was accepted by *Journal of Child Psychology and Psychiatry*. Yet that manuscript has been reprinted in three books including *Annual Progress in Child Psychology and Child Development* (Chess & Thomas, 1974), and it is widely cited. Get an uninvolved friend or colleague to help you interpret any rejection before even considering giving up. Saving your article is very possible.

As we discussed in Chapter 1, the final written version of your research project will not reflect the rich research process you have undergone. It will, however, communicate your ideas and methods to your colleagues and identify you as a resource in the research area you have chosen. Upon publication, you may be surprised at the reprint requests you receive and the letters from other researchers embarking on a related project seeking your advice. Whatever other impact publication has on your career, it earns you a place in a network of scholars working through the imperfect methods of research to build a body of knowledge.

It is quite likely that your research report will end with the usual conclusion: further research is needed. If you have undertaken research in the adventuresome spirit that we have tried to convey in this little volume, we hope that you will be inspired to do that further research.

## SUMMARY

Understanding the findings of the study begins with data analysis. Statistics are only a tool to help in the understanding of data. The appropriate statistics should be kept in mind in designing the study and measures. Initial data analysis includes checking for errors and descriptive statistics. Choosing statistics to test hypotheses depends on the number of variables, the level of measurement, and whether one is interested in measures of association, difference, or predicting group membership.

Communicating findings includes both formal and informal presentations and publication. It is important to consider the audience or audiences who will be interested in the results. Authorship credit is a common source of conflict in large research projects and should be discussed early in the project. Selecting appropriate journals for submission should be done prior to writing the results. Several journals should be selected and a hierarchy of submission constructed in a realistic expectation of rejection. The type of journal, its audience, and its statement of purpose should all be considered. Letters of rejection should be evaluated and should not discourage further efforts at publication. Publication can represent not only the end of the current research project but the beginning of a research program with far-reaching impact.

## EXERCISES

(1) For each of the following hypotheses, specify the two variables of interest and their level of measurement. Does the hypothesis require a measure of association or difference? What statistic would you choose to test it?

   (a) Men who are unemployed are more likely to suffer heart attacks.

   (b) A weight loss program that involves diet and exercise is more effective than one with diet alone.

   (c) The older one is, the higher one scores on Chance Health Locus of Control.

(2) Generate a list of five journals to which you (or someone in your field of study) might submit a manuscript based on research. (This task will probably require going to the library.) What are the differences among these journals?

# REFERENCES

Alexy, W. (1981-1982). Perceptions of ward atmosphere on an oncology unit. *International Journal of Psychiatry in Medicine, 2,* 331-340.

American Psychological Association. (1982). *Ethical principles in the conduct of research with human participants.* Washington, DC: Author.

American Psychological Association. (1983). *Publication manual of the American Psychological Association* (3rd ed.). Washington, DC: Author.

Ardell, D. B., & James, J. Y. (Eds.). (1980). *Author's guide to journals in the health care field.* New York: Haworth.

Baum, A., Gatchel, R. J., & Schaeffer, M. A. (1983). Emotional, behavioral and physiological effects of chronic stress at Three Mile Island. *Journal of Consulting and Clinical Psychology, 51,* 565-572.

Baum, A., Grunberg, N. E., & Singer, J. E. (1982). The use of psychological and neuroendocrinological measurements in the study of stress. *Health Psychology, 1,* 217-236.

Becker, H. S. (1965) Review of P. E. Hammond's sociologist at work. American Sociological Review, 30: 602-603. *Psychology, 1,* 217-236.

Becker, M. H., & Maiman, L. A. (1980). Strategies for enhancing patient compliance. *Journal of Community Health, 6,* 113-135.

Bem, D. J. (1981). Writing the research report. In L. H. Kidder (Ed.), *Selltiz, Wrightsman and Cook's research methods in social relations* (4th ed., pp. 342-364). New York: Holt, Rinehart & Winston.

Bem, D. J. (1986). Writing the research report. In L. H. Kidder & C. M. Judd (Eds.), *Research methods in social relations* (5th ed., pp. 427-451). New York: Holt, Rinehart, & Winston.

Bergman, A., & Werner, R. (1963). Failure of children to receive penicillin by mouth. *New England Journal of Medicine, 268,* 1334-1338.

Bergner, M., Bobbitt, R. A., Carter, W. B., & Gilson, B. S. (1981). The Sickness Impact Profile: Development and final revision of a health status measure. *Medical Care, 19,* 787-806.

Berkman, L., & Syme, S. (1979). Social networks, host resistance and mortality: A nine-year follow-up study of Alameda County residents. *American Journal of Epidemiology, 109,* 186-204.

Bickman, L. (1976). Observational methods. In C. Selltiz, L. S. Wrightsman, & S. W. Cook (Eds.), *Research methods in social relations* (3rd ed., pp. 251-290). New York: Holt, Rinehart, & Winston.

Bliss, R. E., & O'Connell, K. A. (1984). Problems with thiocygnate as an index of smoking states. *Health Psychology, 3,* 563-582.

Bloom, M., & Fisher, J. (1982). *Evaluating practice: Guidelines for accountable professionals.* Englewood Cliffs, NJ: Prentice-Hall.

Boyd, J., Covington, T., Stanaszek, W., & Coussons, R. (1974). Drug defaulting part II: Analysis of noncompliance patterns. *American Journal of Hospital Pharmacy, 31,* 485-494.

Bradley, L. A., Prokop, C. K., Gentry, W. D., Van der Heide, L. H., & Prieto, E. J. (1981). *Assessment of chronic pain.* In C. K. Prokop & L. A. Bradley (Eds.), *Medical psychology.* New York: Academic Press.

Bray, G. (Ed.). (1979). *Obesity in America* (NIH Publication 79-359). Washington, DC: U.S. Department of Health, Education and Welfare.

Brown, G. W., & Harris, T. (1982). Fall-off in the reporting of life events. *Social Psychology, 17,* 23-28.

Cacioppo, J. T., Petty, R. E., & Marshall-Goodell, B. (1985). Physical, social, and inferential elements of psychophysiological measurement. In P. Karoly (Ed.), *Measurement strategies in health psychology* (pp. 263-300). New York: John Wiley.

Cairns, D., & Pasino, J. A. (1977). Comparison of verbal reinforcement and feedback in the operant treatment of disability due to chronic low back pain. *Behavior Therapy, 8,* 621-630.

Campbell, D. T. (1969). Reforms as experiments. *American Psychologist, 24,* 409-429.

Campbell, D. T., & Stanley, J. C. (1963). *Experimental and quasi-experimental designs for research.* Chicago: Rand McNally.

Carmody, T. P., Brischetto, C. S., Matarazzo, J. D., O'Donnell, R. P., & O'Connor, W. E. (1985). Co-occurrent use of cigarettes, alcohol, and coffee in health community-living men and women. *Health Psychology, 4,* 323-335.

Chess, S., & Thomas, A. (Eds.). (1974). *Annual progress in child psychology and child development.* New York: Brunner/Mazel.

Chun, K., Cobb, S., & French, J. (1975). *Measures for psychological assessment: A guide to 3000 original sources and their application.* Ann Arbor: University of Michigan, Institute for Social Research.

Cluss, P. A., & Epstein, L. H. (1985). The measurement of medical compliance in the treatment of disease. In P. Karoly (Ed.), *Measurement strategies in health psychology* (pp. 403-432). New York: John Wiley.

Cohen, J. (1960). A coefficient of agreement for nominal scales. *Educational and Psychological Measurement, 20,* 37-46.

Cohen, J. (1977). *Statistical power analysis for the behavioral sciences.* New York: Academic Press.

Cohen, M. D., March, J. G., & Olsen, J. P. (1972). A garbage can model of organizational choice. *Administrative Science Quarterly, 17,* 1-25.

Cohen, S., Mermelstein, R., Kamarck, T., & Hoberman, H. M. (1985). Measuring the functional components of social support. In I. G. Sarason & B. R. Sarason (Eds.), *Social support: Theory, research and applications* (pp. 73-94). Dordreckt, The Netherlands: Martinus N. Jhoff.

Cohen, W. H. (1985). Health promotion in the workplace: A prescription for good health. *American Psychologist, 40,* 213-216.

Collins, B. E. (1974). Four separate components of the Rotter I-E scale: Belief in a difficult world, a just world, a predictable world, and a politically responsive world. *Journal of Personality and Social Psychology, 21,* 281-291.

Comrey, A. L., Backer, T. E., & Glaser, E. M. (1973). *A sourcebook for mental health measures.* Los Angeles: Human Interaction Research Institute.

Cook, S. W. (1976). Ethical issues in the conduct of research in social relations. In C. Selltiz, L. S. Wrightsman, & S. W. Cook (Eds.), *Research methods in social relations* (pp. 199-249). New York: Holt, Rinehart, & Winston.

Cook, T. D., & Campbell, D. J. (1979). *Quasi-experimentation: Design and analysis issues for field settings.* Chicago: Rand McNally.

Cooper, H. M. (1984). *The integrative research review: A systematic approach.* Beverly Hills, CA: Sage.

Cousins, N. (1979). *Anatomy of an illness as perceived by the patient.* New York: Norton.

Dale, E., & Chall, J. E. (1948). A formula for predicting readability: Instructions. *Educational Research Bulletin, 27,* 37-54.

DeVellis, R. F., DeVellis, B. M., Wallston, B. S., & Wallston, K. A. (1980). Epilepsy and learned helplessness. *Basic and Applied Social Psychology, 1,* 241-253.

Dickson-Parnell, B. E., & Zeichner, A. (1985). Effects of a short-term exercise program on caloric consumption. *Health Psychology, 4,* 437-448.

Dillman, D. (1978). *Mail and telephone surveys.* New York: John Wiley.

Dohrenwend, B. S., & Dohrenwend, B. P. (1978). Some issues in research on stressful life events. *Journal of Nervous and Mental Disease, 166,* 7-15.

Dohrenwend, B. S., Krasnoff, L., Askenasy, A. R., & Dohrenwend, B. P. (1978). Exemplification of a method for scaling life events: The PERI life events scale. *Journal of Health and Social Behavior, 19,* 205-229.

Dohrenwend, B. S., Krasnoff, L., Askenasy, A. R., & Dohrenwend, B. P. (1982). The psychiatric epidemiology research interview life events scale. In L. Goldberger & S. Breznitz (Eds.), *Handbook of stress* (pp. 332-363). New York: Free Press.

Dowling, W. F., & Byrom, F. (1978, summer). Conversation with Fletcher Byrom. *Organizational Dynamics,* p. 43.

Dubbert, P. M., King, A., Rapp, S. R., Brief, D., Martin, J. E., & Lake, M. (1985). Riboflavin as a tracer of medication compliance. *Journal of Behavioral Medicine, 8,* 287-300.

Eichorn, D. H., & VandenBos, G. R. (1985). Dissemination of scientific and professional knowledge: Journal publication within the APA. *American Psychologist, 40,* 1309-1316.

Follick, M. J., Ahern, D. K., & Aberger, E. W. (1985). Development of an audiovisual taxonomy of pain behavior: Reliability and discriminant validity. *Health Psychology, 4,* 555-568.

Fordyce, W. E. (1976). *Behavioral methods for chronic pain and illness.* St. Louis: C. V. Mosby.

Fowler, F. J., Jr. (1984). *Survey Research Methods.* Beverly Hills, CA: Sage.

Friedman, M., & Rosenman, R. H. (1974). *Type A behavior and your heart.* New York: Knopf.

Gellert, E. (1955). Systematic observation: A method in child study. *Harvard Educational Review, 25,* 155-156.

Gordis, L. (1979). Conceptual and methodological problems in measuring patient compliance. In R. B. Haynes, D. W. Taylor, & D. L. Sackett (Eds.), *Compliance in health care.* Baltimore: Johns Hopkins University Press.

Grady, K. E. (1984). Cue enhancement and the long-term practice of breast self-examination. *Journal of Behavioral Medicine, 7,* 191-204.

Grady, K. E., Goodenow, C., & Borkin, J. R. (in press). The effect of reward on compliance with breast self-examination. *Journal of Behavioral Medicine.*

Grady, K. E., Kegeles, S. S., Lund, A. K., Wolk, C. H., & Farber, N. J. (1983). Who volunteers for a breast self-examination program? Evaluating the bases for self-selection. *Health Education Quarterly, 10,* 79-94.

Green, C. J. (1985). The use of psychodiagnostic questionnaire in predicting risk factors and health outcomes. In P. Karoly (Ed.), *Measurement strategies in health psychology* (pp. 301-334). New York: John Wiley.

Grieco, A., & Long, C. J. (1984). Investigation of the Karnofsky Performance Status as a measure of quality of life. *Health Psychology, 3,* 129-142.

Hamilton, M. (1959). The assessment of anxiety states by rating. *British Journal of Medical Psychology, 32,* 50.

Haskell, W. L., Taylor, H. L., Wood, P. D., Schrott, H., & Heiss, G. (1980). Strenuous physical activity, treadmill exercise test performance and plasma high-density lipoprotein cholesterol. *Circulation, 62*(Supp. 4), 53-61.

Haynes, R., Gibson, E., Hackett, B., Sackett, D., Taylor, D., Roberts, R., & Johnson, A. (1976). Improvement of medication compliance in uncontrolled hypertension. *Lancet, 1,* 1265-1268.

Holmes, T. H., & Rahe, R. H. (1967). A social readjustment rating scale. *Journal of Psychosomatic Research, 11,* 213-218.

Holroyd, K. A., Penzien, D. B., Hursey, K. G., Tobin, D. L., Rogers, L., Holm, J. E., Marcille, P. J., Hall, J. R., & Chila, A. G. (1984). Change mechanisms in EMG biofeedback training: Cognitive changes underlying improvements in tension headache. *Journal of Consulting and Clinical Psychology, 52,* 1039-1053.

House, J. S., & Kahn, R. (1985). Measuring social support. In S. Cohen & L. Syme (Eds.), *Social support and health.* New York: Academic Press.

Huck, H. W., & Sandler, H. M. (1979). *Rival hypotheses: Alternative interpretations of data based conclusions.* New York: Harper & Row.

Huskisson, E. C. (1974). Measurement of pain. *Lancet, 2,* 1127-1131.

Jenkins, C. D., Zyzanski, S. J., & Rosenman, R. H. (1979). *Jenkins activity survey manual.* New York: Psychological Corp.

Jick, J. (1979). Mixing qualitative and quantitative methods: Triangulation in action. *Administrative Sciences Quarterly, 24,* 710-718.

Johnson, J., & Leventhal, H. (1974). Effects of accurate expectations and behavioral instructions on reactions during a noxious medical examination. *Journal of Personality and Social Psychology, 29,* 710-718.

Jones, E. E., & Sigall, H. (1971). The bogus pipeline: A new paradigm for measuring affect and attitude. *Psychological Bulletin, 76,* 349-364.

Judson, H. F. (1980). *Search for solution.* New York: Holt, Rinehart & Winston.

Kale, W. L., & Stenmark, D. E. (1983). A comparison of four life event scales. *American Journal of Community Psychology, 11,* 441-459.

Kaplan, R. M. (1985). Quality of life measurement. In P. Karoly (Ed.), *Measurement strategies in health psychology* (pp. 115-146). New York: John Wiley.

Karoly, P. (1985). The assessment of pain: Concepts and procedures. In P. Karoly (Ed.), *Measurement strategies in health psychology* (pp. 461-516). New York: John Wiley.

Keefe, F. J. (1982). Behavioral assessment and treatment of chronic pain: Current status and future directions. *Journal of Consulting and Clinical Psychology, 50,* 896-911.

Keefe, F. J., & Block, A. R. (1982). Development of an observational method for assessing pain behavior in chronic low back pain patients. *Behavior Therapy, 13,* 363-375.

Kelley, A. B. (1979). A media role for public health compliance? In R. B. Haynes, D. W. Taylor, & D. L. Sackett (Eds.), *Compliance in health care* (pp. 193-201). Baltimore: Johns Hopkins University Press.

Kelly, J. R., & McGrath, J. E. (1988). *On time and method.* Newbury Park, CA: Sage.

Kimmel, A. J. (1988). *Ethics and values in applied social research.* Newbury Park, CA: Sage.

Kobasa, S.C.O. (1985). Longitudinal and prospective methods in health psychology. In P. Karoly (Ed.), *Measurement strategies in health psychology* (pp. 235-262). New York: John Wiley.

Kolko, D. J., & Rickard-Figueroa, J. L. (1985). Effects of video games on the adverse corollaries of chemotherapy in pediatric oncology patients: A single-case analysis. *Journal of Consulting and Clinical Psychology, 53,* 223-228.

Krantz, D. S., Baum, A., & Wideman, M. V. (1980). Assessment of preferences for self-treatment and information in health care. *Journal of Personality and Social Psychology, 39,* 997-990.

Kratochwill, T. R. (1978). *Single subject research.* New York: Academic Press.

Kulich, R., Follick, M. J., & Conger, R. (1983, November). *Development of a pain behavior classification system: Importance of multiple data sources.* Paper presented at the annual meeting of the American Pain Society, Chicago.

Langer, E. J., Janis, I. L., & Wolfer, J. A. (1975). Reduction of psychological stress in surgical patients. *Journal of Experimental Social Psychology, 11,* 155-165.

Lavrakas, P. J. (1987). *Telephone survey methods: Sampling, selection and supervision.* Newbury Park, CA: Sage.

Lefcourt, H. M. (1966). Internal versus external control of reinforcement: A review. *Psychological Bulletin, 65,* 206-220.

Levenson, H. (1981). Differentiating among internality, powerful others and chance. In H. Lefcourt (Ed.), *Research with the locus of control construct* (Vol. 1). New York: Academic Press.

Levy, S. M. (1985). *Behavior and cancer.* San Francisco: Jossey-Bass.

Light, R. J. (1971). Measures of response agreement for qualitative data, some generalizations and alternatives. *Psychological Bulletin, 76,* 365-377.

Linkewich, J., Catalano, R., & Flack, H. (1974). The effect of packaging and instruction on outpatient compliance with medication regimens. *Drug Intelligence and Clinical Pharmacy, 8,* 10-15.

Linton M., & Gallo, P. S. (1975). *The practical statistician: Simplified handbook of statistics.* Monterey, CA: Brooks/Cole.

Lipsey, M. W. (1988). *Design sensitivity: Statistical power for treatment effectiveness research.* Newbury Park, CA: Sage.

Martin, J. (1982). A garbage can model of the research process. In J. E. McGrath, J. Martin, & R. Kulka (Eds.), *Judgment calls in research* (pp. 17-39). Beverly Hills, CA: Sage.

Matarazzo, J. D. (1982). Behavioral health's challenge to academic, scientific, and professional psychology. *American Psychologist, 37,* 1-14.

McGrath, J. E. (1982). Dilemmatics: The study of research choices and dilemmas. In J. E. McGrath, J. Martin, & R. A. Kulka (Eds.), *Judgment calls in research* (pp. 69-102). Beverly Hills, CA: Sage.

McGrath, J. E., Martin, J. & Kulka, R. A. (Eds.). (1982). *Judgment calls in research.* Beverly Hills, CA: Sage.

McGuire, W. J. (1973). The yin and yang of progress in social psychology: Seven koan. *Journal of Personality and Social Psychology, 26,* 446-456.

McGuire, W. J. (1983). A contextualist theory of knowledge: Its implications for innovation and reform in psychological research. In L. Berkowitz (Ed.), *Advances in experimental social psychology* (Vol. 16, pp. 1-47). New York: Academic Press.

McQueen, D. V., & Celentano, D. D. (1982). Social factors in the etiology of multiple outcomes: The case of blood pressure and alcohol consumption patterns. *Social Science and Medicine, 16,* 397-418.

Meenan, R. F. (1982). AIMS approach to health status measurement; conceptual background and measurement properties. *Journal of Rheumatology, 9,* 785-788.

Meenan, R. F., Gertman, P. M., & Mason, J. H. (1982). The arthritis impact measurement scales; further investigation of a health status measure. *Arthritis and Rheumatology, 25,* 1048-1053.

Melzack, R. (1975). The McGill Pain Questionnaire: Major properties and scoring methods. *Pain, 1,* 277-299.

Merton, R. K. (1968). *Social theory and social structure.* New York: Free Press.

Micozzi, M. S. (1985). Nutrition, body size, and breast cancer. *Yearbook of Physical Anthropology, 28,* 175-206.

Moos, R. H. (1985). Evaluating social resources in community and health care contexts. In P. Karoly (Ed.), *Measurement strategies in health psychology* (pp. 433-459). New York: John Wiley.

National Cancer Institute. (1979). *Readability testing in cancer communications* (DHEW Publication No. NIH 79-1689). Bethesda, MD: Author.

Nunnally, J. C. (1978). *Psychometric theory* (2nd ed.). New York: McGraw-Hill.

Palinkas, L. P. (1985). Techniques of psychosocial epidemiology. In P. Karoly (Ed.), *Measurement strategies in health psychology* (pp. 49-115). New York: John Wiley.

Park, L. C., & Lipman, R. S. (1964). A comparison of patient dosage deviation reports with pill counts. *Psychopharmacologia, 6,* 299-302.

Parlee, M. B. (1981). Appropriate control groups in feminist research. *Psychology of Women Quarterly, 5,* 637-644.

Peters, T. J., & Waterman, R. H., Jr. (1982). *In search of excellence.* New York: Warner.

Radloff, L. S. (1977). The CES-D scale. A self-report depression scale for research in the general population. *Applied Psychological Measurement, 1,* 385.

Reeder, L. G., Ramacher, L., & Gorelnick, S. (1976). *Handbook of scales and indices of health behavior.* Pacific Palisades, CA: Goodyear.

Reid, J. B. (1970). Reliability assessment of observation data: A possible methodological problem. *Child Development, 41,* 1143-1150.

Rhodes, L. (1981). Social climate perception and depression of patients and staff in a chronic hemodialysis unit. *Journal of Nervous and Mental Disease, 169,* 169-175.

Robertson, L. S. (1975). Safety belt use in automobiles with starter-interlock and buzzer-light reminder systems. *American Journal of Public Health, 65,* 1319-1325.

Robertson, L. S., Kelley, A., O'Neill, B., Wixom, C., Eiswirth, R., & Haddon, W. (1974). A controlled study of the effect of television messages on safety belt use. *American Journal of Public Health, 64,* 1071-1080.

Robertson, L. S., O'Neill, B., & Wixom, C. (1972). Factors associated with observed safety belt use. *Journal of Health and Social Behavior, 13,* 18-24.

Robinson, J. P., & Shaver, P. (1973). *Measures of social psychological attitudes.* Ann Arbor, MI: Institute of Social Research.

Rosenthal, R. (1976) *Experimenter effects in behavioral research.* New York, NY: Irvington.

Rosenthal, R. (1984). *Meta-analytic procedures for social research.* Beverly Hills, CA: Sage.

Rosenthal, R., & Rosnow, R. L. (1969). The volunteer subject. In R. Rosenthal & R. L. Rosnow (Eds.), *Artifact in behavioral research* (pp. 59-118). New York: Academic Press.

Roskam, S. E. (1985). *Health locus of control beliefs in chronic illness.* Unpublished major area paper, Vanderbilt University, Nashville, TN.

Rotter, J. B. (1966). Generalized expectancies for internal versus external control of reinforcement. *Psychological Monographs, 80* (1, whole no. 609).

Rotter, J. B., Chance, J., & Phares, E. J. (Eds.). (1972). *Applications of a social learning theory of personality.* New York: Holt.

Sanders, S. (1980). Toward a practical instrument for the automatic measurement of "uptime" in chronic pain patients. *Pain, 9,* 103-109.

Sandler, I. N., & Guenther, R. T. (1985). Assessment of life stress events. In P. Karoly (Ed.), *Measurement strategies for health psychology.* New York: Wiley.

Schacter, S., & Singer, J. E. (1962). Cognitive, social, and physiological determinants of emotional states. *Psychological Review, 69,* 379-399.

Seligman, M.E.P. (1975). *Helplessness: On depression, development and health.* San Francisco: Freeman.

Sharpe, T., & Mikeal, R. (1974). Patient compliance with antibiotic regimens. *American Journal of Hospital Pharmacy, 31,* 479-484.

Siegel, S. (1956). *Nonparametric statistics for the behavioral sciences.* New York: McGraw-Hill.

Siri, W. E. (1956). *Advances in biological and medical physics.* New York: Oxford University Press.

Skinner, B. F. (1956). A case history in scientific method. *American Psychologist, 11,* 221-233.

Smith, R. L., McPhail, C., & Pickens, R. G. (1975). Reactivity to systematic observation with film: A field experiment. *Sociometry, 38,* 536-550.

Smith, R. A., Wallston, B. S., Wallston, K. A., Forsberg, P. R., & King, J. (1984). Measuring desire for control over health care process. *Journal of Personality and Social Psychology, 47,* 415-426.

Spender, F. W., Corcoran, C. A., Allen, G. J., Chinsky, J. M., & Viet, S. W. (1974). Reliability and reactivity of the videotape technique on a ward for retarded children. *Community Psychology, 2,* 71-74.

Spielberger, C. D., Gorsuch, R. L., & Lushene, R. (1970). *The state-trait anxiety inventory manual.* Palo Alto, CA: Consulting Psychologists Press.

Stanley, K. E. (1980). Prognostic factors for survival in patients with inoperable lung cancer. *Journal of the National Cancer Institute, 65,* 25-32.

Stewart, A. L., Brook, R. H., & Kane, R. L. (1980). *Conceptualization and measurement of health habits for adults in the health insurance study: Vol. 2. Overweight* (R-23742-HEW). Santa Monica, CA: Rand.

Sudman, S., & Bradburn, N. (1985). *Asking questions: A practical guide to questionnaire design.* San Francisco: Jossey-Bass.

Swencionis, C. (1982). Journals relevant to health psychology. *Health Psychology, 1,* 307-313.

Tabachnick, B. G., & Fidell, L. S. (1983). *Using multivariate statistics.* New York: Harper & Row.

Taplin, P. S., & Reid, J. B. (1973). Effects of instructional set and experimenter influence on observer reliability. *Child Development, 44,* 547-554.

Taylor, S. E., Wood, J. V., & Lichtman, R. R. (1983). Selective evaluation of a response to victimization. *Journal of Social Issues, 39,* 19-40.

Terenius, L. Y. (1980). Biochemical assessment of chronic pain. In H. W. Kosterlitz & L. Y. Terenius (Eds.), *Pain and society.* Weinheim: Verlag Chemi.

Timko, C., & Janoff-Bulman, R. (1985). Attributions, vulnerability and psychological adjustment: The case of breast cancer. *Health Psychology, 4,* 521-544.

Turk, D. C., & Kerns, R. D. (1985). Assessment in health psychology: A cognitive-behavioral perspective. In P. Karoly (Ed.), *Measurement strategies in health psychology* (pp. 335-372). New York: John Wiley.

U.S. Bureau of the Census. (1985). *Statistical abstract of the United States: 1986* (106th ed.). Washington, DC: Government Printing Office.

Venham, L., Bengston, D., & Cipes, M. (1977). Children's responses to sequential dental visits. *Journal of Dental Research, 56,* 455-459.

Viet, S. W. (1978). *Naturalistic observation of interpersonal interaction: Methods and models.* Unpublished major area paper, George Peabody College, Nashville, TN.

Wagenaar, T. C. (1981). Social statistics without formulas. In T. C. Wagenaar (Ed.), *Readings for social research* (pp. 281-301). Belmont, CA: Wadsworth.

Wallston, B. S. (1973). Effects of maternal employment on children. *Journal of Child Psychology and Psychiatry, 14,* 81-95.

Wallston, B. S. (1983). Overview of research methods. In B. L. Richardson & J. Wirtenberg (Eds.), *Sex role research: Measuring social change* (pp. 51-70). New York: Praeger.

Wallston, B. S., Alagna, S. W., DeVellis, B. M., & DeVellis, R. F. (1983). Social support and physical health. *Health Psychology, 2,* 367-391.

Wallston, B. S., & Grady, K. E. (1985). Integrating the feminist critique and the crisis in social psychology: Another look at research methods. In V. E. O'Leary, R. K. Unger, & B. S. Wallston (Eds.), *Women, gender and social psychology* (pp. 7-33). Hillsdale, NJ: Lawrence Erlbaum.

Wallston, B. S., Smith, R. A., Wallston, K. A., King, J. E., Rye, P. D., & Heim, C. R. (1987). Choice and predictability in the preparation for barium enemas: A person-by-situation approach. *Research in Nursing and Health, 1,* 13-22.

Wallston, B. S., Wallston, K. A., Kaplan, G. D., & Maides, S. A. (1976). Development and validation of the health locus of control (HLC) scale. *Journal of Consulting and Clinical Psychology, 44,* 580-585.

Wallston, K. A., Maides, S., & Wallston, B. S. (1976). Health related information seeking as a function of health related locus of control and health value. *Journal of Research in Personality, 10,* 215-222.

Wallston, K. A., Smith, R. A., & Wallston, B. S. (1985). *Final report: Effect of patient participation on outcomes* (Research Grant HSO4096). Bethesda, MD: National Center for Health Services.

Wallston, K. A., & Wallston, B. S. (1981). Health locus of control scales. In H. Lefcourt (Ed.), *Research with the locus of control construct* (Vol. 1). New York: Academic Press.

Wallston, K. A., & Wallston, B. S. (1982). Who is responsible for your health? The construct of health locus of control. In G. S. Sanders & J. Suls (Eds.), *Social psychology of health and illness.* Hillsdale, NJ: Erlbaum.

Wallston, K. A., Wallston, B. S., & DeVellis, R. (1978). Development of the Multidimensional Health Locus of Control (MHLC) Scales. *Health Education Monographs, 6,* 161-170.

Ward, M. J., & Lindeman, C. A. (1978). *Instruments for measuring nursing practice and other health care variables* (Publication no. HRA 78-54). Hyattsville, MD: DHEW.

Ware, J. E., Brook, R. H., Davies, A. R., & Lohr, K. N. (1981). *Choosing measures for health status for individuals in general populations.* Santa Monica: Rand.

Webb, E. J., Campbell, D. T., Schwartz, R. D., & Sechrest, L. (1966). *Unobtrusive measures: Nonreactive research in the social sciences.* Chicago: Rand McNally.

Webb, E. J., Campbell, D. T., Schwartz, R. D., Sechrest, L., & Grove, J. B. (1981). *Nonreactive measures in the social sciences.* Boston: Houghton Mifflin.

Weick, K. E. (1968). Systematic observational methods. In G. Lindzey & E. Aronson (Eds.), *The handbook of social psychology* (Vol. 2). Reading, MA: Addison-Wesley.

Weick, K. E. (1981). *The management of organizational change among loosely coupled elements.* Unpublished manuscript.

Woodward, N. J., & Wallston, B. S. (1986). *Age and health care beliefs: Self-efficacy as a mediator of low desire for control.* Manuscript submitted for publication.

Wortman, C. B., & Conway, T. (1985). The role of social support in adaptation and recovery from physical illness. In S. Cohen & L. Syme (Eds.), *Social support and health.* New York: Academic Press.

Wortman, C. D., & Dunkle-Schetter, C. (1979). Interpersonal relationships and cancer: A theoretical analysis. *Journal of Social Issues, 35,* 120-155.

Wyler, A. R., Masuda, M., & Holmes, T. H. (1968). *Journal of Psychosomatic Research, 11,* 363-375.

Yeaton, W. H., & Sechrest, L. (1981). Meaningful measures of effect. *Journal of Consulting and Clinical Psychology, 49,* 766-767.

Zlutnick, S., Mayville, W. J., & Moffat, S. (1975). Modification of seizure disorders: The interruption of behavioral chains. *Journal of Applied Behavior Analysis, 8,* 1-12.

Zonderman, A. B., Heft, M. W., & Costa, P. T. (1985). Does the illness behavior questionnaire measure abnormal illness behavior? *Health Psychology, 4,* 425-436.

Zung, W.W.K. (1971). A-rating instrument for anxiety disorders. *Psychosomatics, 12,* 371-379.

Zung, W.W.K., & Cavenar, J. O., Jr. (1981). Assessment scales and techniques. In I. L. Kutash, L. B. Schlesinger et al. (Eds.), *Handbook on stress and anxiety.* San Francisco: Jossey-Bass.

# AUTHOR INDEX

# SUBJECT INDEX

# ABOUT THE AUTHORS

Kathleen E. Grady is President of the Massachusetts Institute of Behavioral Medicine in Springfield, Massachusetts. She received an undergraduate degree in history from Brown University (1964) and a Ph.D. in social psychology from the Graduate Center of the City University of New York (1977). She did two years of postdoctoral work in health psychology at the University of Connecticut Health Center. Before founding the Institute in 1987, she was Associate Professor in Residence and Acting Associate Dean at the School of Allied Health Professions at the University of Connecticut. Her research activities include several studies on encouraging the early detection of breast cancer, the impact of rheumatoid arthritis on role functioning, and, most recently, AIDS prevention.

Barbara Strudler Wallston was a Professor in the Department of Psychology and Human Development at George Peabody College of Vanderbilt University. She received her undergraduate degree in mathematics from Cornell University (1965) and her Ph.D. in social and personality psychology from the University of Wisconsin (1972). Her research in health and health care was extensive and prolific. She was perhaps best known for the development of the Multidimensional Health Locus of Control Scales with her ex-husband and colleague Kenneth Wallston and others. She was also the author of numerous articles and chapters in the psychology of women and coeditor of the book *Women, Gender, and Social Psychology* with Virginia E. O'Leary and Rhoda K. Unger. She died suddenly in January, 1987.